she
fights
back

ABOUT THE AUTHOR

Joanna Ziobronowicz is a former IBJJF World and European Champion and a black belt in Brazilian Jiu-Jitsu. She was one of the first women to receive a black belt from Roger Gracie.

Combined with her Master's degree at the department of Linguistics and Psychology at University College London and on the ground experience working in security, she brings a much needed and credible voice to women's self-defense.

Joanna uses this platform to empower women as the owner of Women's Self Defense UK, where she works with individuals and corporates to deliver self-defense certification courses and workshops.

She is passionate about serving communities and is an ambassador of REORG charity, who work to improve lives of veterans and emergency services workers through fitness and martial arts.

To find out more, visit www.womenselfdefense.co.uk

she
fights
back

Using Self-Defence Psychology to Reclaim Your Power

WATKINS
1893

She Fights Back
Joanna Ziobronowicz

First published in the UK and USA 2024 by
Watkins, an imprint of Watkins Media Limited
Unit 11, Shepperton House
89–93 Shepperton Road
London N1 3DF

enquiries@watkinspublishing.com

A CIP record for this book is available from
the British Library

ISBN: 978-1-78678-842-9 (paperback)
ISBN: 978-1-78678-844-3 (ebook)

1 3 5 7 9 10 8 6 4 2

Set in Candara
Printed and bound by CPI Group (UK) Ltd, Croydon, CR0 4YY

www.watkinspublishing.com

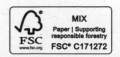

To Lidia,

Let your voice be heard.

ACKNOWLEDGEMENTS

I would like to express my heartfelt gratitude to everyone who has been instrumental in my writing journey.

I want to express my sincere appreciation to Rita for her assistance in shaping the section on martial-arts-related psychology. Her feedback and insights have been invaluable.

I extend my kudos to Sheri for her meticulous review of sections that stretched beyond my academic boundaries. Her words of motivation and support have been a driving force.

Special thanks to Ria for her unwavering encouragement as I embarked on the initial pages of this book.

Last but not least, I want to express my sincere appreciation to JB, whose continuous support has been a constant source of motivation throughout the creative process.

CONTENTS

PREFACE

Congratulations!

You've likely picked this book up to help learn how to create a safer environment for yourself, or for other females in your life. You're about to embark on an empowering journey of discovering how caution and preventative measures are crucial in avoiding conflict, and how they can be used as a first line of defence. You will also learn what to do in emergency situations.

You may relate to some of the stories, as I'm sure you have some of your own to tell. As well as my own accounts, I also share various anecdotes from clients, students, friends and co-workers, with some of the names anonymized for privacy purposes.

I hope that the voices of the women who have shared their stories with me will inspire and motivate you. My wish is that the tools and narratives provided in this book will help you to recognize your own strengths and connect you to your inner warrior spirit, so that you, too, are ready to stand up and fight back.

INTRODUCTION

I find myself lying face down on the ground, my sweat dripping onto the floor. With my waistline immobilized, I tightly grip the arm that's pressing against my neck, fighting to free myself from the strangle. I can't hear anything; it's as if a continuous radio sound wave is beaming into my ears. I'm gasping for air, feeling my eyes becoming bloodshot and starting to close, and my face is throbbing from the tension. Repeating the mantra to breathe and focus, I execute the survival steps in a flawless sequence. With determination, I bridge my hips vigorously, moving my legs to the side, and with that, I manage to release myself from the hold.

The timer rings, signalling the end of the round.

My training partner smiles as we shake hands, expressing gratitude for the exchange.

Some people would interpret this as a harrowing moment to live through. For others, this scenario embodies courage, and could be viewed as one of life's most empowering moments. Overcoming a struggle can be incredibly impactful, and can present us with an opportunity to unearth our inner warrior heroine.

This book is all about her – the empowered female who uncovers the psychological and physical strengths within herself, nurturing them to stay confident, bold and authentic, taking charge, and passionately safeguarding her values and her personal safety.

* * *

As children, we are often told stories about good prevailing over evil, and about that elusive "happily ever after". As little girls, we may be taught that if we're obedient, we will be rewarded for our goodness. When we grow up, some of us realize that always conforming and always being kind can threaten our boundaries, shatter our sense of self-worth, and at times, expose us to trauma.

I wouldn't be writing this book if I myself hadn't fallen victim to detrimental cultural conditioning, psychological trauma and physical attacks that I had to overcome. It took many years and many uncomfortable life lessons to cultivate a strong sense of self-belief, as well as to acquire the valuable physical skills needed to protect myself, but these experiences were necessary in helping me understand what women need to do to keep themselves safe.

After years of working in the security sector, I've learned that in addition to relying on my martial arts skillset, it is also crucial to stay alert and keep a watchful eye over people and surroundings.

When I was working in security, threats could come from anyone and anywhere, often when I least expected them. All it took was one moment of inattention to be caught off guard. However, over time, I found common patterns and warning signs that allowed me to spot and assess threats early on, leading to more efficient responses.

By watching my work colleagues handling conflicts, and also by getting involved in various physical interventions myself, I came to realize that some of the most critical aspects of self-defence are having confidence in your own abilities, and having conviction in your actions. I noticed that these qualities were primary drivers for performance, and for finding solutions when faced with highly triggering situations. Today, I know that I could teach you how to impeccably execute the most effective self-defence moves, but without the ability to assert yourself and without self-belief in your capabilities, they won't be enough.

I observed similar psychological aspects of performance during my sports career, both as a coach and as an active competitor in various martial arts. With over 23 years of training experience, I have seen that high performance is fuelled by incredibly strong self-belief, unwavering conviction, and a razor-sharp mindset. I've studied alongside world-class athletes, have competed at the highest level, and time and time again I've demonstrated, both to myself and those that I coached, that everything begins in the mind. I've seen exceptionally talented athletes freeze before tournaments, mentally giving up before even setting foot into the competition arena. I've learnt that a champion is made not just through appropriate physical preparation, but also through a strong mental drive toward their actions and achievements.

With this in mind, we should explore both the physical and psychological aspects of self-defence. If you want to win your battles, it's time to acknowledge and build upon the confidence that will enable you to assert your rights, stand up for yourself, and stay physically prepared.

* * *

I have written this book with the hope of empowering every woman who is concerned about her safety in this modern world. In this era of digital information, reporting and statistics, we now have more evidence than ever before to help us understand the nature of threats that exist in our everyday lives. Through anonymous surveys and government data, there is ample proof to demonstrate that violence against women is, unfortunately, still very common.

According to the World Health Organization, one in every three women globally experiences violence during their lifetime, either as physical and/or sexual intimate partner violence or as non-partner sexual violence. This is a disturbing statistic, but one that can be changed.

My goal is to reveal the nature and origin of the most common threats, and to offer pre-emptive measures, tools and solutions to boost women's awareness, confidence and assertiveness. This book focuses on reinforcing the mental aspects of our female power – alongside the physical ones – in order to prevent these threats from harming us. The book will demonstrate how to use emotional intelligence, how to de-escalate conflicts, and how to employ various psychological and linguistic techniques to address challenging situations. I draw examples from my personal experience, from my work in the security sector, as well as from my academic background and further research.

Additionally, this book offers guidance on how to use and strengthen your body in order to improve your chances of defending yourself against physical attacks. It introduces ten key physical strategies to address common scenarios, and offers suggestions on defensive steps and escape tactics for each situation.

Last, but certainly not least, this book also provides strategies for coping with assault-related trauma.

Please note that some of the content discussed in this book is of a sensitive nature, and may be triggering. It is my heartfelt wish to expose these difficult topics to the light, so that they don't get shoved onto the shelf of taboos, but rather are explored with kindness and compassion. In this way, we can find the strength to overcome our struggles, and empower ourselves to make positive changes going forward.

CHAPTER 1
WOMEN'S POWER

"You have power over your mind – not outside events. Realize this, and you will find strength."
—Marcus Aurelius

Amy grabs Lily's hand as the latter blushes with intimidation, having forgotten what she was supposed to do. Amy, a complete stranger to Lily, calms her down and guides her to perform the move correctly. Lily tries again and stops halfway through. She hesitates. I come over and reassure her, telling her that she must not give up. She must keep trying until she succeeds. Five minutes later I come back around, and this time, Lily's new partner, Katy, encourages Lily to perform the same move with her eyes closed. Lily pauses, adjusts her posture and shuts her eyes, allowing her training partner to grab her. She repeats the same movement until the grip breaks, pointing her hands at Katy, moving a couple of steps back, working her de-escalation tactic. I congratulate her on executing the move correctly. She smiles and her eyes water with joy. She is ready to go again.

What Lily experienced in this moment was a level of self-confidence and self-belief that she had not felt in a long time. Her surging emotions were reinforced by other females in the room, filling her with optimistic collective feedback. With the realization that there is no competition between them, the women at the workshop enact the roles of fellow participants, rather than the roles of attackers and defenders. The real fight taking place on the mat is the one within themselves, deep down, facing their own fears and insecurities.

Once the thread of mutual recognition is repeated, with the same positive reinforcement, something magical takes place in that space and time. A rebirth of self-belief, built upon other women's encouragement and drive. This phenomenon, drawing from the collaborative action, is something that is present across all groups, regardless of different social backgrounds, ethnicities and ages. Embarking on a mission to rediscover themselves, women fuel each other's desire to build their own inner strength and confidence.

For some, it will come more naturally than for others, as we practise verbal and physical role play. At times, when a woman finds it difficult to access her female warrior spirit, I encourage her to imagine a vivid scenario in which someone she loves is being threatened. This simple visualization changes everything, as she will instantaneously summon the strength of a giant. Her body language changes. Her voice becomes clearer, her eyes sharper, and her chest more open. Sometimes she will raise her voice to share what she would do to the perpetrator. She becomes a Valkyrie, deciding on who will live and who will get punished.

Something quite incredible happens in these moments, and it is something that science is only just beginning to understand. There is a mental, but also a physical strength that builds within the female body – and the relentless and invincible warrior woman spirit is being released. The psychological part of the warrior woman is now ready to fight, and her physical body follows suit.

The warrior woman knows that protecting herself and her loved ones is the only thing that really matters. She throws off the cover of "compliant participant" and is ready for battle. Just like Jennifer Lopez in the movie *Enough*, she breaks through, ready to fight.

Each workshop becomes a reminder of that nearly forgotten female power that lies deep within each of us, ready to be unveiled. The rekindled feminine fire I witness in each seminar is a testament to the fact that we're all capable of taking action, and of accessing the force to fight for what matters the most. In terms of personal safety, this will mean everything from setting expectations, boundary protection, de-escalation, right up to the last resort – physical action.

Unlocking Women's Power: The Reality of Self-Defence

When asked to conduct self-defence workshops, people often expect me to demonstrate flashy moves, resembling those of Steven Seagal, that could incapacitate any man, regardless of his shape or size. Just imagine how impressive it would be to break a man's wrist with just one strike, leaving him paralysed and begging for mercy. Unfortunately, these things only happen in movies. Similarly, women often envision violence from strangers as being just as it is portrayed in the media – men lurking on dark street corners. These images have little to do with everyday life, and everything to do with making you feel anxious and in need of a preventative quick fix. So, let's get back to planet Earth and detangle the true meaning of primary defence mechanisms, which can help us tap into our women's power and protect us from danger.

There are two main components of being a powerful woman – psychological strength and physical strength. They are often intertwined, as our mental aptitude drives physical confidence, and vice versa. Understanding how we can draw from both of these forces can help us formulate the best responses and reactions when faced with situations that we fear the most – when our values are undermined, our boundaries are threatened and when our personal safety is at risk.

Firstly, in the "psychological dojo", we'll delve into the topic of "good girl conditioning", to discover how women have been programmed to desire acknowledgement and acceptance, and to enact certain roles in society. We will see how growing up abiding by certain rules and behaviours can create barriers to valuing and protecting our own inner experience, and how this can contribute to non-existent or denied boundaries, and an inability to express anger. By bringing to light various elements of this phenomenon, we will explore ways in which we can break free from good girl conditioning, starting with asserting and protecting our boundaries, and learning how to communicate them effectively in everyday situations. We will also examine what happens when we enter the psychological state of "freeze", and will look at how to change the power dynamic in a verbal exchange. These methods will be paramount for establishing a stronger sense of control when dealing with difficult situations, and can make us better communicators.

Apart from addressing the disadvantages associated with being a woman, we will also explore the ways in which we can tap into our female power and enhance our strengths, which in turn will boost our self-esteem and confidence. We will discuss which skills and activities can improve our assertiveness and help us feel more in charge during conflict. Additionally, we'll also discover how to employ our intuition and emotional intelligence to deal with disputes and conflicts. We will observe ways in which we can learn and practise those skills.

In the physical dojo, we will unravel three components of talent in order to determine how we can build new skills in the most effective way. We'll also briefly discuss the mood-boosting qualities of hormones released during physical activity.

In the Strengths Assessment exercise, we will take note of where we currently stand in terms of our skills and abilities.

Finally, we will discuss the future of our young females, and how we can collaboratively work towards improving the lives of women through education and training.

Psychological Dojo

Breaking the Good Girl Conditioning

Good Girl Jail is the socio-psychological (and sometimes very real) prison in which many women find themselves today: trapped, stifled, bound by the limiting norms of "Good" in a patriarchal society. Approved Good Girl behaviours have been so well learned, rewarded and perpetuated amongst both men and women for millennia, that Good Girl conditioning is so normalized you'd be forgiven for thinking it was innate, even biological.[1]

Good girl conditioning is something that comes up a lot in various cultures. Societal pressure for women to act in a certain way isn't yet a thing of the past, even though some would like to believe that it is. In many traditional households, women still fall into the role of quiet, abiding conformists. It is usually through the university of life that we discover that this type of conditioning is not conducive to creating clear and healthy boundaries in the modern world.

The behaviours of good girl conditioning are internalized from a young age. It is a collective insistence upon women that they please other people, at the cost of their own wellbeing. It's the moulding of a female into behavioural patterns which are deemed appropriate. Clinical psychologist and author, Dr Nicole LePera, explains that good girl conditioning is messaging we receive, beginning in childhood, to be

---

1   www.kasiaurbaniak.com/blog/the-good-girl-jailbreak

9

agreeable, polite and nice. To "never show our anger, to allow people to violate our boundaries and to hide our own needs to please others. Young girls who take on these traits are rewarded in families as well as society."[2]

LePera explains that being good very often comes with a price. By neglecting our boundaries, we become unable to express ourselves, and as a consequence, many young women fall into the freeze state, or a "fawn trauma" response. In the freeze state, we are often unable to speak, our minds "frozen", and in the fawn trauma response, we become overly compliant to avoid danger, harm or inconvenience.

An example of how this can play out is often seen during social interactions and gatherings, where family members impose a certain type of behaviour on a young female. Imagine a situation where, as a young girl, you're in the presence of a revolting and intoxicated uncle whom you're afraid of. Your mother recognizes your feelings of discomfort, yet proceeds to urge you to remain polite. Perhaps you're asked to give your uncle a kiss, or a cuddle, as your tummy starts to churn. Have you experienced a similar scenario in the past?

Perhaps you recall a situation in which you disrupted a conversation, took up space or expressed your opinion, and got reprimanded for it? Did you feel ashamed, curling into a cocoon of unacknowledged feelings and needs? Many women have certainly felt this way, as we have been primed to sacrifice our wellbeing to please others – to keep things on an even keel.

This dynamic of neglected and unacknowledged emotions replays itself to the point where we start to become disconnected from our own feelings, denying and devaluing our own experiences. As the cycle of denied emotions is repeated, just imagine the impact that this type of conditioning will have on future adult interactions, when honouring and respecting your

2   twitter.com/Theholisticpsyc/status/1587223722804453376

boundaries is impossible, and you freeze when faced with a disorderly or menacing individual.

It's worth noting that it's not solely societal pressure that creates good girl conditioning behaviours in women. In the fascinating book by Robin Norwood, *Women Who Love Too Much*, the author explores the topic of girls who are brought up in disturbed households and become conditioned to take on the roles of silent observers. Living in an unstable or threatening environment (for example, living with an alcoholic), females learn not to cause trouble and to never ask for anything. They remain quiet, not wanting to add any burden to the family or the situation. The good girl "blends into the wallpaper, says very little. ... as for her own pain, she is numb, she feels nothing".[3]

This conditioning caused by growing up in disturbed households can also reveal itself in future romantic relationships, where women "tend to believe that suffering is a mark of true love, that to refuse to suffer is selfish, and that if a man has a problem, then a woman should help him change".

Norwood makes a great point about how women can easily fall into the trap of taking on a carer role. This usually happens when a young female observes the sacrifices of her own mother, then takes on the same mission to save everyone else, at the cost of her own wellbeing. This can have disastrous consequences when it comes to a woman valuing her own experience, honouring her boundaries, and respecting her needs. What it often leads to is engagement in toxic and abusive relationships with a partner who exploits the woman's vulnerabilities. This is the scenario we see in the vast majority of male assaults on women, where female domestic abuse victims suffer in silence, subconsciously taking on the victim role in the relationship. The only way out of this loop, and to prevent victimization in the first instance, is to seek help. With the appropriate

3   Norwood, R, *Women Who Love Too Much*, Arrow Books, 2004

support, a traumatized woman can start to dismantle the mechanisms of abuse, and begin to learn strategies to reaffirm her values and her sense of self-worth.

* * *

Another feature of good girl conditioning is being told (directly or indirectly) to never show anger. The good girl is taught that being angry comes across as rude and inappropriate. She learns how to avoid, deny or bottle up that feeling. Perhaps you, too, grew up in a household where anger was shamed and criticized? If you had an abusive parent, then you may have learnt to supress anger as a coping strategy, to avoid danger.

The problem with pushed-down anger is that it can result in the tendency to try to avoid conflict, creating difficulties during confrontation and in setting boundaries. You may find it difficult to stand up for yourself, or to say no to other people. This could also lead to self-sabotage and lowered self-esteem. The good girl suffering from supressed anger will find it very difficult to cope in threatening scenarios, or when her boundaries are violated. She will sit still in the corner, freeze, and very often say nothing. Experiencing anger may come with a feeling of shame, or even guilt, adding more reasons to repress the emotion. As we subconsciously avoid it, it sits in the shadows, only to reveal itself upon deeper self-reflection, or therapy work.

One way in which we can start to recognize our own anger is through its manifestations in the body. Observing our physical reactions can be revealing, and can help us to spot anger when it emerges. In a stressful situation, you can tune into your body and notice everything you're experiencing. Observe reactions such as a tight chest, a headache, increased heart rate, feeling hot, sweating (especially in the palms), trembling, or feeling dizzy. The body's reaction can be a helpful way of identifying that you may be experiencing anger. Try and tune into these feelings, rather than avoiding them. It's important to recognize the sensations and give them space, while becoming confident in your power to deal with the reactions. This way, you will be able to spot anger without giving it control, yielding the incessant need to conceal and supress it.

Once you're able to recognize the manifestations of anger in your body, acknowledge and give it space, the next step will be to learn how to release your anger safely. While there are many strategies, a great way to let out anger is by getting physically active. Any form of sporting activity can be beneficial. For some, this may be cardiovascular training, such as jogging, or cycling. For others it may be through lifting weights. Transmuting anger into something physical will bring about a better sense of control and stability, and through emotional regulation you'll be able to stay on top of situations that are triggering and scary.

*   *   *

In order to protect yourself from any form of victimization, it's important to acknowledge which area of good girl conditioning you currently find yourself in. Perhaps you have uncovered a tendency to reject anger, or maybe you have felt the urge to be unnecessarily polite and to never come across as rude. Maybe you have noticed feelings of discomfort when expressing your boundaries, or asserting your needs.

If these suggestions do not resonate with you, think about other day-to-day scenarios.

For example, have you been afraid to ask for a raise, been anxious when returning a dish at a restaurant, or felt unease when declining an offer or a proposal?

If you find yourself identifying with any of these examples, then you too have fallen into the good girl conditioning trap! While healing from these programmed behavioural patterns can be a lifelong process, Dr Nicole LePera offers a few suggestions to help us get started. Some of these include:[4]

- Setting boundaries
- Understanding your needs and communicating them
- Honouring your emotions
- Avoiding over-explanations.

In the next section of this chapter we'll dive into the area of boundaries, defining what they are and how to best protect them. We will explore how boundaries help us to value ourselves and our experiences, and how this can be crucial in preventing unwanted and violent behaviour.

Assessing and Protecting Boundaries

When I discuss boundaries, I like to recall a situation from the days when I worked in the security sector. I use this story to help students understand that even the most inconspicuous woman has the power to protect her physical and personal space.

The situation occurred at a night club in West London, with music buzzing and people wobbling with intoxication. Our security eyes, as always, were laser sharp, trying to determine when and where another culprit might initiate a drunken brawl. As I scanned the club, I noticed a small Latina woman, about five foot tall, push a big man across the bar, then slap him across the face so hard a vibration was sent across the room. The man froze in utter shock. The woman pointed a finger at him, shouting that he was to never touch her "booty" again. As the male doormen intervened, I stood in awe of what this woman accomplished. With her warrior spirit, she sent a groper home in the most humiliating way

---

4 LePera, N, *How to Do the Work: Recognize Your Patterns, Heal from Your Past, and Create Your Self*, Harper, 2021

possible. She stood there looking bold, appearing taller than she actually was, as she made herself visible by taking up space and opening up her body in a winner-like fashion.

In that moment, this woman took a calculated risk, doing what she deemed was appropriate in order to protect her boundaries. She reacted not only by making a scene, but also by physically engaging with the man to expose him as a harasser. While the use of physical force may not have been substantiated, the level of risk of him retaliating was relatively low.

When deciding how best to protect your boundaries, it is crucial to appropriately assess the situation and then act proportionally. At the end of the day, what matters is that we go home safe, without risking any potential consequences for our actions.

The process of assessing and implementing boundaries can be divided into the following stages:

- Defining boundaries
- Communicating boundaries
- Setting consequences.

Defining Boundaries

The first step to understanding boundaries is to do a personal assessment of what they mean for us individually. We need to know what our boundaries may look like at work, in personal relationships and during interactions with strangers. Recognizing and acknowledging our boundaries will be an important tool for personal safety, as this will help determine when and how to clearly set expectations for ourselves and for others. Our boundaries will be protective shields with the power to ward off situations in which our mental and physical wellbeing may be at risk.

Boundaries will also vary from person to person, and it is crucial for you to establish your own based on your own experience and moral compass.

You may find that you discover your personal boundaries through the school of hard knocks. Observing your reactions and triggers can also be helpful to determine where on the spectrum of acceptance certain behaviours and actions lie for you. This will vary depending on the social context in which these behaviours appear. For example, it's perfectly acceptable for your partner to show you affection, while it may not be acceptable for a work colleague to do so.

Communicating Boundaries

The second step in implementing boundaries is that we need to be able to convey our wishes, needs and expectations in a straightforward and honest way. If you have been programmed to be the good girl, then you may find that after communicating your boundaries, you feel discomfort, guilt or shame. Acknowledge that this is a natural part of breaking out of the good girl conditioning. Do not let these feelings stop you from continuing to assert your needs. When practising boundary setting in a non-violent environment, we can remain calm, direct and assertive. There is no need to raise your voice, as we can communicate our wishes simply, clearly and concisely. On the other hand, when our personal and physical space is being threatened, this changes the way we should approach boundary assertion. In that circumstance, our voice can become more audible, and statements can be made in a more precise, definitive and dominant manner.

Setting Consequences

Setting consequences for the breaking of boundaries can be very helpful in terms of personal safety. When being threatened, you should alert the perpetrator to the consequences of their actions. You can mention the level of support that you will get when reporting them to the appropriate authorities, or people in charge. This strategy could be put in place against anyone who is behaving in a disorderly manner: from an inappropriate work colleague or a supervisor, to a street harasser or an online stalker.

In the following exercise, you will ask yourself questions about the social contexts in which your boundaries may be threatened, and set out a plan on how to best communicate and protect them. Tapping into the feelings associated with boundary assertion will prepare you for taking appropriate action in the future. Practising this type of boundary defence on a daily basis will condition you to become a better communicator of your needs and expectations.

EXERCISE: SETTING BOUNDARIES

For both your personal and professional life, list two needs or boundaries which you would like to work on. When stating what they are, describe the feelings associated with both having and not having achieved them. How will you communicate these feelings? Verbally? By text? What words will you use? Can you picture/visualize the experience?

If you need more space, you can write your answers down in a separate notebook.

Example

Personal boundary/need: I need my boyfriend to stop shouting at me.
Feeling experienced when achieved: Relief, tranquillity, trust.

Feeling experienced when not achieved: Agitation, anger, fear, panic, resentment.

How will I communicate my feelings?: Face to face in a quiet space, I will slowly and calmly explain how shouting affects me emotionally and physiologically.

* * *

Personal boundary/need: ....
....

Feeling experienced when achieved: ....
....

Feeling experienced when not achieved: ....
....

How will I communicate my feelings?: ....
....
....

Personal boundary/need: ....
....

Feeling experienced when achieved:...............................
....

Feeling experienced when not achieved: ....
....

How will I communicate my feelings?: ....
....
....

Professional boundary/need: ....
....

Feeling experienced when achieved:...............................
....

Feeling experienced when not achieved: ....
....

How will I communicate my feelings?: ....
....
....

Professional boundary/need: ....
....

Feeling experienced when achieved:...............................
....

Feeling experienced when not achieved: ....
....

How will I communicate my feelings?: ....
....
....

If you start this exercise on a Monday morning, at the end of the week, you should reflect on how things are going with your boundary goals by completing the following three sentence stems:

In order to keep working on this boundary or need, it may be helpful to ....

....

....

In order to keep working on this boundary or need, it may be helpful to ....

....

....

In order to keep working on this boundary or need, it may be helpful to ....

....

....

(The sentence stem approach has been adapted from Nathaniel Branden's clinical methodology on improving self-esteem.[5] For the full set of comprehensive exercises on boundaries, review the author's book *The Six Pillars of Self-Esteem*,[6] or visit his official website.)

---

5   Branden, N, "Sentence Completion I", https://nathanielbranden.com/sentence-completion-i/
6   Branden, N, *The Six Pillars of Self-Esteem*, Bantam, 1995

Take Aways

- The process of boundary setting can be divided into three stages: defining boundaries, communicating them, and setting consequences.
- Boundaries are very individual and largely depend on the context in which they appear.
- With time and experience, you have the opportunity to observe and learn from your reactions and triggers to determine where your boundaries currently lie.

Changing the Power Dynamic in a Verbal Exchange

Now that we have delved into the topic of good girl conditioning, let's think about how we can set something very powerful into motion: changing the power dynamic in a conversation.

The act of practising how to change the power dynamic can help us in our psychological dojo, and when dealing with stressful situations, difficult people and the unexpected in general.

In her book *Unbound*, author Kasia Urbaniak explains that for centuries, women have been taught to keep their attention on themselves – putting them in an inward state of attention, thus assuming the submissive state. As a result, when presented with a problem or a difficult situation, women can enter a state of freeze. Urbaniak's interpretation of the state of freeze refers to a psychological state in which we are devoid of ideas – we enter "neuromuscular lockdown" in which we "cannot speak, or worse", find ourselves "nodding yes – implying consent and agreement when in fact you're desperate to say no".[7]

When you find yourself in a psychological state of freeze, rest assured there is a way out. As Urbaniak explains, in order to flip the power dynamic, you need to turn your attention

---

7   Urbaniak, K, *Unbound: A Woman's Guide to Power*, Vermillion, 2021

outward. When you are put on the spot, or put in a situation where you feel like you're being forced into a submissive state, switch the attention back to the person who currently dominates the conversation. By turning the attention back onto the speaker, by putting *them* in the spotlight, you are moving yourself into the dominant position, and forcing *them* to turn inward for a moment.

In the dominant position, you're ten times more likely to walk out of the room. You're fifty times more likely to stand up for yourself. And you're a hundred times more likely to say no when you mean no.[8]

When you are asked a difficult or rude question, and find yourself in a state of freeze, Urbaniak proposes a simple strategy – ask a question back. Following this advice, when someone enquires, for example, about your age or marital status, you can simply reply by saying, "Are you sure you want to ask me that question?" or, "Is this an appropriate question to ask a woman during an interview?"

Asserting your position does not have to come across as angry or aggressive. It can be handled in an intelligent yet firm way, when you surprise your "opponent" by asking them a question instead of answering theirs. This puts you in charge, and puts them in the spotlight. If you are someone that doesn't naturally ooze confidence, this technique can quickly and effectively put you out of the victim role and into a state of dominance.

Turning the power dynamic is something that works really well in a self-defence workshop during role play, when we practise assertiveness skills. I often instruct women to assume the dominant role in a conversation where they are not sure what to do or what to say. When approached by

---

8   Urbaniak, K, "Can't Speak Up? It's Not a Lack of Confidence. It's the Freeze", https://www.kasiaurbaniak.com/blog/women-with-confidence-break-the-freeze

a colleague acting as a stranger, the role of the "target" is to take space with her body language, and take control by picking the correct verbal response. This practice is always by far the hardest exercise for most women in the room, as they start to recognize how they have been conditioned to freeze. For most of the women, assuming a dominant posture and thinking of a strong verbal response suddenly feels like an impossible ask.

While not every situation will be straightforward to handle, nor possible to tackle by just asking a question, the simple technique of changing the power dynamic can be extremely helpful in breaking social conventions and turning the seemingly submissive female roles into dominant ones during a difficult interaction. The one who owns the conversation holds the power, and as Urbaniak explains, when used in the right place at the right time, this can save us from falling into the trap of good girl conditioning. This will allow for healthier relationships, more focused boundary assertions, and the protection of ourselves and our wellbeing in general.

EXERCISE: REWRITE THE SCRIPT

In this exercise, try to recall situations during which you have fallen into the state of freeze, or when you noticed good girl conditioning at play. Remind yourself of what was done or said that triggered you. Disregard your verbal responses or reactions at the time.

Instead, flip the script and rewrite the experience, stating what you are going to do now.

Visualize each scenario as clearly as you can, naming the feelings present (whether supressed or not), noticing your body language, and recognizing the boundary being threatened. Remain as detailed as possible, as this will help restructure your reactions, and tap into the empowered version of yourself.

Once in a quiet space, after writing down your reactions, practise them in front of a mirror. Take ownership of your feelings. You can replay this scenario as many times as you like, to the point where it feels natural and exudes confidence.

If you find it difficult to recall particular stories from your past, imagine situations that could potentially occur in your workplace, or in your personal life, in which you may feel threatened or triggered. Pre-emptively craft the ideal response using the following example that is provided.

If you need more space, you can write your answers down in a separate notebook.

Example

Situation: Boss asked me if I was happy with my boyfriend.
Emotional reaction: I feel uncomfortable, ashamed, frozen, taken by surprise.
Physical reaction: Head turned down, blushing, hands fidgeting.
Verbal reaction: Mumbled something quietly, can't even remember exactly what I said.
Value/boundary being threatened: Privacy, integrity, ethics.

Rewriting the script: I take charge of the conversation by turning the attention onto the speaker, and asking them a question back.
Emotional reaction: I tap into the anger. How dare he ask me this question?
Physical reaction: I force myself to look him in the eyes, taking space but remaining poised.

Verbal reaction: I ask him, "Surely, this is not the topic we are here to discuss?"

* * *

Situation 1: ....
....

Emotional reaction:. ....
....

Physical reaction: ....
....

Verbal reaction:.. ....
....

Value/boundary being threatened: ....
....

Rewriting the script: ....
....

Emotional reaction:. ....
....

Physical reaction: ....
....

Verbal reaction: ....
....

Situation 2:...

....

Emotional reaction:. ....

....

Physical reaction:. ....

....

Verbal reaction: ....

....

Value/boundary being threatened:. ....

....

Rewriting the script:...

....

Emotional reaction:. ....

....

Physical reaction:. ....

....

Verbal reaction: ....

....

Boosting Self-Esteem and Confidence

As we have seen in the examples of good girl conditioning, at times, societal norms and traditions can programme us in ways which aren't always conducive to creating healthy relationships, or a strong sense of self. Some of us will not have noticed the unhealthy patterns and broken boundaries until we experience heartbreak from a toxic relationship, a painful divorce, or until we find ourselves on a therapist's couch, opening the emotional Pandora's box for the first time. Like a scientist dissecting a body, we seek to determine the root cause of our predicament, eventually to stumble upon the topics of self-esteem and self-worth.

We discover that self-esteem is not only about being confident about our own worth and abilities, but is also about being responsible for ourselves, our actions, our feelings and our needs. Self-esteem is crucial when establishing boundaries, and protecting oneself as a woman. Without self-esteem, we become more vulnerable to manipulation, grooming, and psychological and physical abuse. The lack of self-esteem is bound to attract violent partners, and staying in abusive relationships will further reinforce the idea that we are not worthy of guarding ourselves from harm.

*   *   *

While there are a multitude of ways in which we can strengthen our self-esteem, I have witnessed one in particular that has a long-lasting impact on females, and that is the practice of self-defence.

In a study conducted at the University of Washington, where 80 college students aged 18–23 underwent a six-week self-defence training course, it was found that the course boosted the level of self-esteem amongst the women and positively affected their personalities. The coauthor of the study reported that women who completed the course felt more assertive and less hostile and aggressive. One of the authors explains that:

> Skills are important, but so is the perception that you have the skills to take care of yourself. What may be the

most valuable lesson these women learned is not the expertise they picked up – like how to break a choke hold or kick someone in the knee – but the knowledge that they have the skills to keep a situation from escalating into violence and, if necessary, protect themselves.[9]

In the self-defence courses I deliver, the most common feedback relates to the psychological impact of the workshops. Students report feeling empowered and more confident, and less anxious to face future conflicts.

For some of the women attending a self-defence course, it's the first time in their lives that they acknowledge their skills and what they are capable of. They discover that within themselves lies the power to change the outcomes of many situations, enabling them to employ strategies to control and prevent conflicts. They observe their bodies being capable of doing much more than they previously believed possible. This newfound skill and belief can prove invaluable when dealing with conflicts, taking defensive action, and standing up for themselves in times of trouble.

* * *

Another way to boost confidence is to get involved in a new hobby or to learn a new skill. In the psychological dojo, activities that involve communication and problem solving can be extremely helpful. Often, this means stepping out of your comfort zone, where you have to employ new strategies and learn how to thrive in an unknown environment. A great example of this is public speaking, something many of us dread and associate with sweaty palms, an increased heart rate and panic. However, public speaking doesn't have to

---

9 Schwarz, J, "Learning Self-Defense Teaches Women Far More Than Just How to Protect Themselves, It Kick Starts Self-Esteem", *UW News*, www. washington.edu/news/1997/08/12/learning-self-defense-teaches-women-far-more-than-just-how-to-protect-themselves-it-kick-starts-self-esteem/

mean performing in front of a large audience. Expressing oneself in front of others and engaging in conversations with new people is one way to embrace a smaller challenge and to practise building your assertiveness. As uncomfortable as it may seem, it will be incredibly valuable.

Stepping out of your comfort zone is one of the most rewarding strategies to deepen the perception of psychological strength. By consistently immersing ourselves in situations that aren't pleasant or agreeable, we condition ourselves to deal with discomfort. The more we engage in scenarios that scare us, the more opportunities we have to practise managing our emotions. As we become confident in our capabilities, it translates into a deeper sense of control and power.

The more skilled we become in facing conflict with emotional stability, the less likely we are to enter the state of freeze. As the freeze state can completely paralyse us, making us unable to act, it's important that we nurture a sense of self-belief, so that when difficult scenarios arise, we are able to deal with them more successfully.

To practise facing adversity, regularly schedule time when you can step out of your comfort zone. If you're not currently experiencing any significant challenges at work or in your personal life, I recommend engaging in activities that can push you just beyond your comfort zone. This will allow you to experience dealing with unease while having the capacity to positively reframe it, reminding yourself that you've just moved out of your bubble and that you're bound to feel unstable.

Having an accountability partner in crime is also a great idea, as you can share the experience with someone who can support and motivate you. In Chapter 2: Cultivating Confidence, we explore various activities and exercises that can further assist you in exploring your confidence and boosting your self-esteem.

Take Aways

- Self-esteem is having confidence in your worth and abilities, but also being responsible for yourself. It's crucial for boundary assertion and when protecting yourself.
- Lack of self-esteem can lead to attracting violent partners and abusive relationships.
- One way to positively boost confidence and the feeling of self-esteem is by engaging in new activities and hobbies. These could include martial arts training and self-defence, as well as any new activities that can challenge us physically and psychologically.

Accessing Your Female Power

Have you ever been in a vulnerable situation and quite unexpectedly managed to handle it? Perhaps in an important exam, a job interview, a difficult discussion with your boss, or maybe when facing an angry or threatening individual?

Mel, one of my clients, recently shared a story about being on a night out with her friends, when an intoxicated stranger approached her, put his arm around her shoulder, and mumbled flirtatiously at her, inviting her to dance. Mel, naturally shy and easily intimidated, felt repelled by the smell of alcohol on the man's breath, a reminder to her of her abusive ex-boyfriend. She found herself firmly placing her palms against the man's chest, forcefully pushing him away, and warning him that she would call security for help. Mel did not recognize herself in that moment – she was driven by deep emotion and the fear of getting hurt. She tapped into an invisible force, that of a protective warrior spirit.

I once found myself in a similar situation, when two inebriated men on a bus were speaking Polish, not realizing my language comprehension. One of the men fired appalling comments in my direction, delivering an instant dose of adrenaline into my nervous system. I found myself entering a very charged state, sensing my heartbeat beginning to race and my palms getting sweaty. As the bus slid up to the curb, I grabbed the abuser's shirt, pushed him against the bus window, and in his native language served him a *Pulp Fiction*-sounding verbal throw back. The man bolted upright in utter shock as his colleague apologized for the inappropriate behaviour, ushering his friend to the exit door. Seconds later, the men vacated the bus, and I took a seat to process what had happened, feeling like the warrior princess Xena returning from battle. In that moment, just like my client Mel, I experienced a feeling of being taken over by a strange force erupting from within, fuelled by indignation and anger.

Have you experienced this state before? If you have, you know that once we tap into our inner fire, there is very little that can stop us. We are capable of accessing strength within us that is so powerful, both physical and mental barriers seem non-existent. Just as Angela Cavallo released her son (who was trapped under a car) by lifting a vehicle with what is referred to as "hysterical strength", many a woman can tap into her fearless warrior spirit. In this state, we are ready to fight for our safety, we are ready to fight to protect our lives and the lives of others, and we are ready to fight for our dignity.

In the following exercise, I encourage you to reflect deeply on your past experiences, to see when and where you were able to access your inner strength. Remind yourself of situations that triggered you, and think of the reasons and emotions that fuelled you into action.

EXERCISE: REMEMBER YOUR STRENGTH

Remind yourself of moments in your life when you tackled a stressful situation or took action, even though you felt scared. Maybe you challenged your boss, a street stalker, or took charge when someone threatened you.

Name the situation, the feelings you experienced during the confrontation, and your feelings once the situation was resolved. What was it like to tap into your female warrior spirit? How did your body feel? Did it make you feel more powerful and confident? Did it boost your self-esteem?

If you need more space, you can write your answers down in a separate notebook.

Situation 1:. ....

Feelings during confrontation (what fuelled you?): ....

....

....

Feelings once the situation has been resolved:. ....

....

....

Situation 2:. ....

Feelings during confrontation (what fuelled you?): ....

....

....

Feelings once the situation has been resolved:. ....

....

....

Tapping into the Female Intuition

If you have ever wondered whether or not it is a myth that women are better at reading people then men, you may find the answer in a recent study conducted by Cambridge University, in collaboration with researchers from Harvard, Washington, and other universities. In order to gather enough evidence, over 300,000 people were involved in the study.[10]

In the test, participants were asked to pick words that best described the thoughts or feelings being experienced by a person shown in a photo, by viewing their eyes. The skill of being able to read such feelings and emotions is often referred to as "theory of mind" or "cognitive empathy". Unsurprisingly, the study proved that women, on average, were better at reading facial expressions and emotions than men. Across the 57 studied nations, there wasn't one country in which males scored more highly than women.

This means that women are better at picking up on subconscious cues than men. It may also explain why women tend to report having gut feelings about certain people more often than men do. The feeling may manifest itself in different ways, and in order to learn how to recognize it, we need to remind ourselves of situations where we experienced certain feelings or sensations.

For example, do you recall having a recurring knot in your stomach when meeting certain individuals? When dating, I experienced this more than once, and it was most apparent with dates that happened at a meal time, when I felt as if my stomach was being "locked". It wasn't until years later that I learnt these bodily reactions were prompts about my safety in a particular environment, rather than gastric

---

10 Greenberg, D M, et al., "Sex and Age Differences in 'Theory of Mind' Across 57 Countries Using the English Version of the 'Reading the Mind in the Eyes' Test", *Proceedings of the National Academy of Sciences of the United States of America*, vol. 120(1), 2023, e2022385119. doi:10.1073/pnas.2022385119

problems. After all, in the company of a different person on the same day, I could easily wolf down a meal with taste and pleasure. Needless to say, none of the dates accompanied by this negative gut feeling ended successfully. Which was a relief, as the nagging sensations were certainly not pleasant to experience!

These subconscious signs and feelings, such as the tingling in the gut, don't just pertain to strangers. A belly cringe can also be experienced when spending time with an acquaintance, or a family member. Here again, boundaries and listening to the voice of intuition may prove crucial when deciding whether to object, resist or leave. Saying "no" to someone within our circle, especially when they hold a position of power and authority, does not come easily. The same goes for young female adolescents, who are only beginning to learn about consent, and are prone to experience coercion in various social contexts, including with their peers. What is imperative to note is that when a female is faced with a sexually motivated pursuit, the gut feeling is most potent. In his book *The Gift of Fear*, author Gavin de Becker goes over numerous interviews with victims of sexual violence as they explicitly report having experienced gut feelings before being sexually assaulted.

We are all equipped with this fabulous gift from mother nature. Learning how to use it correctly can give us power beyond our rational minds, and can protect us from danger.

You may ask yourself, how come we so often ignore it?

The reason we are quick to disregard our intuitive signals is that we are largely driven by our neocortices and cognitive processing, which guide us in the decision-making process. We have strayed away from our connection with nature, and have learnt to heavily rely on tangible, palpable data. We have also learnt to question and distrust ourselves.

The real problem lies in the fact that most of us have lost the deep connection to the feelings and emotions that run through us. We don't know how to read them, and sure enough, we are not ready to embrace them with an analytical eye. We cringe with discomfort, deny and reject our own inner experience. We don't recognize the ailments that come in the form of psychosomatic explosions of bottled-up emotion, buried resentment, unresolved traumas and chronic stress. Becóming more attuned to our sensations, emotions and triggers, we can start to recognize and interpret the signs our bodies are handing us on a silver platter.

To practise connecting to our inner experience, we can introspectively meditate, or use therapy-based approaches for more self-reflective work. We can also dissect the feelings by asking ourselves questions when we experience them, to determine whether we are having a gut feeling, or reliving a past experience.

So how do we discern intuitive thoughts and trauma-related anxiety? The key here is to learn the history of how our stress responses and traumatic experiences manifest in the body. Being able to recognize the wounded child within us will make us more attuned to the emotional reactions associated with trauma.

Differentiating between a trauma response and a gut feeling in a situation of high-level risk does not always come easy, but the voices will vary slightly.

Trauma responses can trigger:

- A lack of steadiness
- A sense of imbalance
- Preoccupying feelings flooding the body, coming in like fire.

According to Victoria Albina, a trauma response:

is jangly, it is scratchy and urgent, harried and rushed. It's future tripping or spinning in the past. It's an analysis paralysis. Spinning you 1,000 ways from Sunday. It doesn't quite know which way is up, but it sure does know you're not doing it right. It's worked up and needs you to listen, right now. It's spinning. Never still.[11]

Gut feelings:

- Are alert, firm and loud
- Provide a sense of clarity that comes with a sense of knowing
- Speak in a loving, non-judgemental way.

Intuition, according to Albina:

is the gentle singsong tone of voice that I have ... the safe and social, present and connected, part of the nervous system. It's inviting, versus coercive.

Take Aways

- The fact that women are better at "people reading" has been proven in studies.
- Listening to the voice of intuition may be especially helpful in social contexts when we interact with people.
- Gut instinct usually manifests as a tingling in the belly, or a knot in the stomach.
- In order to be able to discern between instinctive reactions, and trauma-related anxiety, we need to be able to understand our past history, our reactions and triggers.
- The voice of intuition varies slightly from trauma-related triggers, as it manifests in the sensation of knowing, and being alert, as opposed to feeling imbalanced and "scratchy".

---

11 Albina, V, "Ep #201: Your Intuition Vs. Trauma", *Victoria Albina*, victoriaalbina.com/intuition-vs-trauma/

Employing Emotional Intelligence

I was working a night shift in one of the biggest clubs in London when we received a radio request to remove a disruptive, drunken customer. This typically meant that two doormen, one on each side, would physically hold the individual to escort them out. This time I decided to take up the challenge, eager to test my negotiation skills and to see whether the customer would respond differently to a female. Deep down, I was quite possibly also keen to assess the effectiveness of my jiu-jitsu skills in real life.

Off I went, wearing an oversized black hoodie, looking unassuming but prepared to face the intoxicated individual. As I touched his wrist, I looked him in the eyes and asked him to follow me. To my surprise, the man smiled politely and zigzagged his way to the elevator. I couldn't believe his compliance and my luck as the lift took us to the ground floor. He looked perplexed when he was handed over to my colleagues waiting by the exit door, and once he realized his predicament, it was too late, as there was no alternative route to get back in.

As humorous as this situation was, it showed me that I could employ similar tactics for situations which normally would require physical prowess and potential altercation. Here I was, ready to wrestle, in what turned out to be the easiest customer ever to be taken out of the club. Until the next obedient one, who I politely ushered to the elevator the next day, in the same exact fashion.

I tell this story often, mostly because it's fun to hear, but also because it is such a great example of how females can try strategies that use the path of least resistance.

Sometimes this will involve trickery (like in this example, where I wasn't upfront about the fact that I was removing the customer from the club), or by employing more intricate emotional intelligence strategies, which can be extremely helpful for women, as they don't involve physical intervention.

* * *

Considering the fact that women score higher on emotional intelligence tests than men,[12] it makes us great candidates to use this skill. But what exactly is emotional intelligence?

Emotional intelligence is the ability to manage our emotions in times of stress, but it's also the skill of being able to communicate effectively in order to diffuse conflict. It is a practical tool used by females working in education, hospitality, care units and emergency services. The often empathetic and caring nature of women allows us to handle situations in a non-violent manner, resolving conflicts through verbal communication and de-escalation.

During my interview with Freya, a female police officer from Berkshire, she emphasized the central role of communication in her approach to resolving conflicts.

Freya recalled a story from her early days in the police force, when she was tasked with searching a male who was aggressive and resistant. She noticed needles sticking out of his pockets as he thrashed around, making it challenging to restrain him.

Freya's approach was to maintain a calm yet assertive tone of voice. She believed that a more aggressive approach could have resulted in the man becoming more agitated and angry. She explained her intentions, what she was looking for, and what the man needed to do in order for both of them to walk away from the situation safe and unharmed. She also explained the consequences if he didn't allow her to fulfil her duties. Rather than jumping into a physical altercation, Freya made sure the male understood his options and recognized that she would confidently manage whichever route he decided to take. The man cooperated and disclosed where

12 Brackett, M A, Mayer, J D, Warner, R M, "Emotional Intelligence and its Relation to Everyday Behaviour", *Personality & Individual Differences*, vol. 36, 2004, pp. 1387–402.

he had hidden the needles, allowing Freya to conduct the search without getting hurt.

Physical intervention or application of force was not necessary in that situation, as Freya chose to employ strategies such as risk assessment, maintaining calmness and emotional control and using steady body language, combined with wise and confident communication.

A similar account was shared by Elaine, a current female police officer. She recounted an incident where she received a call about a high-risk individual who had been reported missing after leaving the hospital with suicidal intentions. The patient was described as being a very muscular male with aggressive tendencies. When Elaine arrived on the scene, she noticed the man was surrounded by five other male police officers who were drawing Tasers, as he aggressively threatened to hurt them. Having gathered feedback about the man's past (history of post-traumatic stress disorder from his time in the forces) Elaine decided to intervene, taking a different approach.

Elaine believed that in order to get through to the individual, she had to change the energy of the situation from aggressive and fearful, to something that would calm the man down. She walked up to him, putting her hands up in a passive gesture to denote a peaceful approach. As she drew closer to him, she told the man that she also had been in situations that left her vulnerable, and assured him that she was not speaking solely from a police officer's perspective, but rather from a human perspective.

As she managed to establish a rapport with the man, she gestured for her colleagues to step back, trying to build trust. She understood that the presence of male officers was escalating the aggression, so she engaged in a one-on-one interaction with the man, giving him space to manage his emotional turmoil while she remained calm and empathetic. Eventually, she successfully persuaded the individual to return to the hospital for further assessment of his mental health.

In Elaine's example, emotional intelligence was the key to success, as she effectively resolved a seemingly threatening situation in a calm and efficient manner.

Recognizing when to apply emotional intelligence is a skill which can be developed through experience. It involves learning to assess risks, combining reason with instincts, managing emotions, and communicating effectively. These strategies are interwoven in the psychological dojo, as they all serve as effective tools when dealing with conflicts and encountering threatening scenarios.

Physical Dojo

Components of Talent

While some of us might have a genetic edge when it comes to physical strength or build, those of us in the fitness coaching field quickly learn that genetics is just one piece of the puzzle. Confidence, cardiovascular fitness, and dexterity are skills that develop through experience and training. There's no magic formula here; it's all about staying consistent.

Likewise, in the world of martial arts, inborn qualities don't get you very far if you're not willing to put in the hard work and stay focused. There's solid evidence to support this perspective. In the eye-opening book *The Talent Code*, by Daniel Coyle,[13] the author explains how talent is something that's cultivated, not something we're born with. Coyle draws from neuroscience and research to illustrate how what is commonly referred to as "talent" is actually nurtured and developed.

---

13 Coyle, D, *The Talent Code: Greatness Isn't Born. It's Grown. Here's How,* Bantam, 2009

According to Doyle, the key components of talent include deep practice, ignition and master coaching. These principles apply whether you aim to become a skilled athlete, linguist or musician. They help you stay focused, to mentally handle stress, and to physically prepare for challenging situations. If you aspire to become a strong and powerful female, in control of yourself and your environment, let's explore the three ways you can make it happen.

Deep Practice

The first component of talent is deep practice. This involves targeted repetition with intense focus. It is performed at the edge of your ability, meaning that you're capable of doing it, but it pushes you beyond your current limit. In the physical self-defence dojo, this means going beyond your area of comfort. Examples of this can include practising with strangers, with your eyes closed, and under controlled tension which will be increased over time. In those specific moments, you will break through your current state of knowledge and experience a transformation into a more powerful version of yourself.

Ignition

The second stage of improving talent is ignition. In our dojo, this would be the primary motive – a wish or aspiration to start a training routine, or to sign up to a workshop. This could be built from our deep desire to protect ourselves and our loved ones. If you can tap into whatever it is that you passionately believe in, you can find a motivation strong enough to drive your actions. For a lot of my students, ignition often stems from fear – the fear of being attacked after an assault story on the news, or the fear of future victimization following a recent attack. Can you find what your ignition may be?

Master Coaching

The third component of talent development is what is referred to as "master coaching".

A coach is needed in order to fuel the passion, to inspire the individual and to bring the best out of them. This component is so often disregarded as we strive to perfect ourselves, in our own inner dojos, with self-help books and online programmes. And while all of these are great, in order to set yourself in the right direction and to progress as a disciple of the pursuit you want to work on, you need a mentor – a power figure that will break you to make you.

Take Aways

- Consistency should be your top priority when building your strengths.
- Deep practice, ignition and master coaching are essential elements for building talent.
- The components of talent can apply to any pursuit you choose, whether it's taking self-defence classes or mastering communication skills.

The "Feel Good" of Exercise

Whichever sports discipline you choose for yourself, it's likely to strengthen you inside and out. From feeling more confident in your body, having time to engage with others, or being more physically adept – there are a plethora of benefits that come with physical training.

Apart from the elements already mentioned, such as boosting self-esteem, engaging in fitness activities can also improve your mood, and there is ample research to prove it. Certain hormones produced in our bodies are released during exercise, and a lot of them have mood-boosting qualities. Some of these hormones include:

Dopamine – Known as the "feel-good" hormone, dopamine is an important part of the reward system associated with pleasant feelings. Dopamine can help relieve depression and make us experience joy. It can also aid in repairing the neurological changes that can happen through substance abuse. While we naturally lose some of our dopamine receptors with age, which may lead to us feeling less enjoyment in our daily lives, we can help to control this decline with physical activity.[14]

Serotonin – This mood-stabilizing hormone is associated with feelings of happiness, and helps to control appetite, sleep, libido and digestion.[15] It also influences our learning and memory. Lack of serotonin is linked to depression and anxiety, among many other health conditions.

Oxytocin – The so-called "love hormone", released through exercise, helps promote trust, empathy and bonding. It can also reduce stress, blood pressure and cortisol.[16]

Endorphins – Possibly the most talked-about hormones associated with fitness activities, endorphins offer natural pain relief. Endorphins can lower stress and improve our mood and overall wellbeing.

In order to see the mood-boosting rewards of physical activity, you should seek activities that are either moderate or intense in their nature. Moderate activity would be

14 McGonigal, K, *The Joy of Movement: How Exercise Helps Us Find Happiness, Hope, Connection, and Courage*, Avery, 2019
15 Berger, M, et al., "The Expanded Biology of Serotonin", *Annual Review of Medicine*, vol. 60, 2009, pp. 355–66. doi:10.1146/annurev.med.60.042307.110802
16 Petersson, M, Uvnas-Moberg, K, "Oxytocin: A Mediator of Anti-stress, Well-being, Social Interaction, Growth and Healing", *Zeitschrift fur Psychosomatische Medizin und Psychotherapie*, vol. 51(1), 2005, pp. 57–80. doi:10.13109/zptm.2005.51.1.57

anything during which you can observe your breathing quicken, while still being able to hold a conversation. Some of these activities can include outside walks, dancing, biking, swimming, hiking, vacuuming or mowing the lawn. It's usually recommended that we do 30 minutes of moderate activity on most days, mixing some of those moderate activities with more demanding physical tasks wherever possible.

Bearing in mind that our psychological health is closely linked to our physical health, the benefits you reap through getting active are endless. When you are feeling more empowered, motivated, joyful, and less stressed, you can start to recognize your unique skills and abilities, and to positively reframe any negative beliefs which may have held you back.

Strengths Assessment

A group of women gather in a self-defence workshop, arriving barefoot on the tatami mats. I guide the group to form a circle, and as they huddle together, we introduce ourselves. It's time for some ice breakers, and I ask the ladies if they have past experience with sports and fitness. I notice many heads shaking "no". I dig a little deeper, naming common childhood games and activities such as tree climbing, baseball and ice skating. A few heads start to nod, and all of a sudden, the group's energy becomes more lively as they reminisce about family hikes, playing ball with their kids, or taking part in dance contests years ago.

We all have our backgrounds and things we're good at, but it's quite common for women to underestimate their own experience, often doubting their own skills and abilities. Sometimes, it takes a bit of soul-searching to realize that you might have physical and psychological strengths that you've lost sight of. In this journey of female warrior exploration, it's time to drill down into each area of your life – personal, work, family and social interactions – to rediscover some of these forgotten strengths. You may discover that you excel in some areas, while recognizing that there's still room for growth in others. The following exercise will determine which physical and mental strengths you can recognize in yourself.

EXERCISE: STRENGTHS ASSESSMENT

Please rate yourself on a scale of 1 to 5, with 1 being the weakest and 5 being the strongest, in each of the following categories listed.

Psychological Dojo

Protecting boundaries	① ② ③ ④ ⑤
Verbal communication	① ② ③ ④ ⑤
Confidence and self-esteem	① ② ③ ④ ⑤
People reading	① ② ③ ④ ⑤
Emotional intelligence	① ② ③ ④ ⑤
Gut feeling/intuition	① ② ③ ④ ⑤

Physical Dojo

Cardiovascular fitness	① ② ③ ④ ⑤
Endurance (intensity over time)	① ② ③ ④ ⑤
Physical strength	① ② ③ ④ ⑤
Balance and coordination	① ② ③ ④ ⑤
Reflex/speed	① ② ③ ④ ⑤
Flexibility	① ② ③ ④ ⑤

Now that you have a clear picture of where you stand on each of these scales, you can easily identify your strengths, as well as your areas for improvement. In the next chapter, we'll dive deeper into the practices that can help you boost all of these aspects, so that you can channel your inner female warrior even more. When you revisit this section in the future, recognize any improvements you've made in the mentioned strengths and re-evaluate them as needed.

The Future is Female

The future is female, and it is up to us how we pave the way for future generations of women. With the warrior spirit to influence us, we can fill a new chapter on the pages of female empowerment. We can change the narrative of what it means to be a woman, by collectively taking charge of the roles that we play in our society, and by helping those who need us the most – younger women.

Young females are the most vulnerable group, susceptible to peer pressure, manipulation and abuse. According to WHO, teenage girls between the ages of 15 and 19 are the group most affected by violence from their intimate partners.[17] Just imagine experiencing violence at this age! Nearly a quarter of these girls will have been physically, sexually or psychologically abused by the time they reach their 19th birthday, but that's only the tip of the iceberg, as many cases go unreported.

In the US, nearly 80 per cent of female sexual assault victims report their first assault before the age of 25.[18] A

17 World Bank, "Violence Against Women and Girls – What the Data Tell Us", *The World Bank Gender Data Portal*, 2022, genderdata.worldbank.org/data-stories/overview-of-gender-based-violence/
18 Kuadli, "32 Shocking Sexual Assault Statistics for 2023", *Legaljobs*, 2023, legaljobs.io/blog/sexual-assault-statistics/

similar statistic has been reported in the UK, where women between the ages of 16–24 were more likely to be victims of sexual assault than women over the age of 25.[19] The most vulnerable group, unsurprisingly, were students.

With these staggering statistics, it's apparent that protecting boundaries without compromise should be a topic of discussion in every school and university, as these are some of the places where the threat of female physical and psychological abuse is greatest.

As cruel as the statistics are, there is not only hope, but also a track record of proof about which educational methods work. We have strong evidence for how targeted programmes used in schools and universities can empower young females and decrease their chance of victimization.

In a research study done by the Sexual Assault Resistance Education (SARE) centre, published in the *New England Journal of Medicine*, we see a 46 per cent reduction in completed rape and a 63 per cent reduction for attempted rape for the group (of first-year female university students) that took part in the Enhanced Assess, Acknowledge, Act Sexual Assault Resistance programme, as compared to the control group (who did not take part in this anti-assault programme) in the subsequent year.[20] Other variables, such as non-consensual sexual contact, were also reduced significantly in the group that took part in the programmes. These findings are truly profound, as this study, which was conducted on a group of 893 women, clearly reveals a solid course of action for helping to prevent abuse among female students.

The teachings used in the study's anti-abuse programme are what should stand at the core of every female self-defence course. In the first instance, it puts focus on resistance, which

19 Crime Survey for England and Wales, 2020
20 Senn, C Y, et al., "Efficacy of a Sexual Assault Resistance Program for University Women", *New England Journal of Medicine*, vol. 372(24), 2015, pp. 2326–35, doi:10.1056/NEJMsa1411131

represents the attitudes of and actions taken by women to refuse to accept or comply with social norms or expectations. The resistance could stand for anything, from protecting boundaries, to protecting the body, to sexual integrity when interacting with other people.

The programme focuses on preventing acts perpetrated by men who are known to women, including acquaintances, family members, intimate partners, classmates, neighbours and so on. This topic helps demystify the commonly held belief that sexual violence is usually committed by complete strangers. This allows women to recognize that threats often come from people they know, helping them to become more attuned to risk detection involving non-stranger violence.

The data proves that coercive behaviour is something that can be recognized through proper education, and that can be tackled effectively by recognizing and protecting one's values and boundaries. It's clear that through supportive education, we can become stronger in our convictions, decisions and actions.

* * *

While there is still much to be done in terms of education, the empowered female warrior spirit is ever-present. Its dormant nature can be brought to light by other females. It can be revealed by going through shared experiences. It can also be awakened with appropriate training, and through the power of collective action and discourse.

If we want to see the change, we need to take action. The best thing you can do for young females is to get them involved in educational and physical programmes. Certain types of training are extremely helpful when building confidence, and when paired with appropriate coaching, they can positively boost young women's self-esteem, making them more assertive and open to challenges. If you work in education, launching a female sexual assault prevention programme or female self-defence course in your institution is likely to bring about the best results.

In my years of teaching, I've had the pleasure of working with teenagers and young women who, thanks to their training, were able to display remarkable courage when faced with challenges. One story that truly touched my heart involved one of my youngest students. After completing a self-defence course, she fearlessly confronted a stranger on the bus who was behaving inappropriately. She told him to stay away, and the adults in the vicinity stepped in to protect her. She later shared that she had learned this assertiveness tactic in our course, which inspired her to take action when the situation called for it.

If you are looking for confidence-boosting and authentic self-defence disciplines for yourself or your children, consider the level of physical contact present in your chosen sport – the more contact the better. While most fighting arts instil discipline, condition the body, and teach resiliency, some are more realistic for learning self-defence than others. Examples of fighting sports that encourage close-range physical contact include judo, Brazilian jiu-jitsu and wrestling.

Other examples of popular combat sports such as boxing, kick-boxing or Thai boxing can help develop long-, middle- and close-range blocking and striking tactics, but don't involve breakaway techniques or ground defence.

Take Aways

- Protecting boundaries without compromise is something we learn as we grow. With the correct education, we can decrease the number of sexual violence cases among young females.
- Studies prove that self-defence training positively boosts self-esteem and confidence.
- The best preventative education is the type of

training where females are able to build on both their psychological and physical strengths.

- Most martial arts and combat sports positively boost confidence, condition the body and instil discipline, but for realistic self-defence, consider disciplines that include close-range physical contact such as judo, Brazilian jiu-jitsu, wrestling, kick-boxing or Thai boxing.

Conclusion

We are all powerful women. Whether we believe it or not, the female warrior is present in each and every one of us. In the past, we may have been conditioned to take on the roles of rule-abiding puppets. We may have struggled to break through old-fashioned societal constructs. But we all have the power within us to take on fearless action, to advance and grow in unprecedented ways, and to disrupt the obsolete narrative of what it means to be a woman.

We have the capacity to love and care, but also to be bold and authentic. Once we tap into the strengths within us, there is little that can stop us. With the correct tools in place, we can begin to respect our boundaries without the need for building walls around us. We can start to trust those who deserve our trust, and we can also learn how to trust ourselves, our gut feelings and our emotions.

We can inspire each other as women, young and old, moving together toward a brighter and better future – one in which women are protected and understood.

CHAPTER 2
CULTIVATING CONFIDENCE

Tools for a Strong Body and Mind

"Life is not easy for any of us. But what of that? We must have perseverance and, above all, confidence in ourselves."

—Marie Curle

Andria was on her way home in West London when she noticed a couple of young boys loitering around in the street near her apartment. With an iPad in her hand, she confidently walked past them, noticing their unsteady body language and curious looks. Out of the corner of her eye, she saw one of the boys rushing toward her, as he proceeded to snatch the device. In a firm voice, she told the boys to step back, ready for a potential physical confrontation. Andria affirmed her stance, secured a steady grip on the iPad, then vigorously pulled it back toward her chest. She managed to retrieve the iPad from the boy's grasp, and the two youngsters quickly ran off behind the apartment building.

Andria's success in this situation didn't stem from just one facet of her character, but rather from a range of confidence-building tools that led to a quick and appropriate response. She was aware, not only of herself, but also of those around her. She maintained her composure and effectively problem-solved, making a deliberate decision on how to react. Both her verbal and non-verbal cues were on point, and her body showed readiness for a potential conflict. Andria's mental state played a significant role in her body's reactions. She remained calm, maintaining a strong focus. Even with her heart racing and her body reacting to stress, she didn't let extreme emotions take over. She continued to breathe and stay present.

The confidence toolkit employed by Andria is something that we're all capable of implementing, as it can be built up over time. In this chapter we will go through each one of those tools to help you understand what they are and how you can practise them.

First, we'll explore mindfulness, and discuss techniques that can help us achieve a balanced state of mind, improving focus, stability and awareness. We'll also discuss mastering effective verbal and non-verbal communication, using specific exercises to strengthen our voice and body language. We'll cover fun practices like role play, rehearsals and power poses for gaining confidence and assertiveness. Additionally, we'll take a look at Imago Dialogue, to learn strategies for handling conflicts and building better understanding with others. In addition to psychological and communication tools, we'll get into various forms of physical training to see how this can prepare us for unexpected situations. We'll also explore ways to prevent traumatization through martial arts and self-defence training.

Mindfulness

The first confidence tool that deserves attention, and which is key to successful understanding of the self, is mindfulness. Deeply ingrained in various religious practices from Hinduism to Buddhism, mindfulness is a type of meditation that allows you to focus on and be aware of your sensations and feelings in the present moment, without interpretation or judgement.

Mindfulness has been largely popularized by western schools of yoga as the practice expanded into secular traditions and non-religious methodologies. Various mindfulness-based programmes have also evolved over the years, including Mindfulness-Based Stress Reduction (MBSR) and Mindfulness-Based Cognitive Therapy (MBCT) for the treatment of major depressive disorder.

For those who practise it regularly, mindfulness offers numerous benefits, many of which can be seen in situations that would otherwise cause increased levels of stress, and pose threats to our safety. By practising mindfulness, we can develop a heightened awareness of the present moment, and foster objectivity toward our thoughts and emotions. This, in turn, can assist us in maintaining a sense of calm composure, ultimately improving our ability to focus and concentrate.

* * *

To understand mindfulness, you can begin with yoga, meditation, or specific mindfulness practices. In the following section, I will present a few simple mindfulness exercises that can help you get started.

When considering mindfulness practice, please keep the following points in mind:

- Consistency is more important than the duration of the practice itself. Aim for regularity to establish the habit, ideally on a daily basis. Setting a specific time of the day to practise mindfulness can also be a good option if you prefer routine.
- Begin with shorter sessions, lasting between five to ten minutes each, to make it more manageable, and then gradually increase your practice time.
- Experiment with different times and locations to find out what works best for you.

EXERCISE: MINDFULNESS PRACTICES

In the following mindfulness meditation examples, the goal is to focus on experiencing sensations and feelings in the present moment, without judgement or interpretation.

Attentive Observation

Observe your environment using all your senses: touch, sight, sound, smell and taste. Next time you have a meal, try to sense the texture, smell and taste of the food you are having. When you go for a stroll, observe what it feels like to walk on the ground, noticing everything around you, from the moss on the ground to the different patterns on the leaves. Allow the act of observation to occur naturally, resisting the temptation to name anything. Try to spend at least one minute each day focusing intently on an object or the surrounding environment. You can repeat this practice as many times as your day allows.

Body Scan Meditation

Find a quiet place where you can stay uninterrupted for a few minutes, with your cell phone switched off and as few distractions from the outside world as possible. Ideally, this would be a space where you feel comfortable and at ease. Create a relaxed and peaceful environment using whatever elements you find conducive. For example, you can lie down in a resting position on your back, with your hands and legs extended and palms facing up. Relax your gaze or close your eyes completely. Focus on each part of your body, starting from your forehead, working all the way down to your toes. Pay attention to any sensations or emotions you may be experiencing.

Mindfulness Breathing Meditation

Begin by finding a comfortable seated position, either on a cushion or a yoga mat, with your legs crossed and your back straight. It's beneficial if your hips are positioned above your knees, as this can help alleviate any tension in the back. To allow this, you can place a pillow underneath you. Alternatively, you can sit on a chair with your feet parallel and grounded on the floor, allowing your hands to rest on your thighs or in your lap.

Gently close your eyes, or focus your gaze softly at a point in front of you.

Find the natural rhythm of your breathing, taking easy and relaxed inhales and exhales. Connect with the sensation of the breath as it enters and leaves your body. Observe the rise and fall of your chest and belly with each inhale and exhale.

You may notice that your mind starts to wander. Simply acknowledge it without judgement, then guide your attention back to your breath. In order to achieve more focus, observe each inhale and exhale. Keep the same count on every inhale and exhale, for example breathing in and out on the count of four, or keeping each inhale and exhale on the count of six. Gently pause on the top and bottom of each breath. Notice any subtle changes in your body that occur during this process.

As you practise, cultivate a sense of ease and kindness toward yourself, recognizing that thoughts will naturally arise and pass. Approach your experience with curiosity rather than judgement. Continue breathing for few minutes, and when you are ready to conclude this practice, gently open your eyes, allowing yourself a moment of conscious awareness to acknowledge how you feel in your body.

Another incredibly helpful breathing practice which will allow you to calm down your nervous system is the parasympathetic breathing method. We will discuss this technique in Chapter 4: Facing Conflict in the context of threatening scenarios, but it can also be practised daily to reduce stress, lower heart rate, and promote relaxation.

Take Away

• Mindfulness as a meditative practice is an important confidence tool, as it allows a person to achieve a state of calmness and focus, which contribute to a better sense of control when faced with difficult or stressful scenarios.

Visualization for Inner Strength

Many successful people throughout history, including athletes such as Michael Jordan, Muhammad Ali and Billie Jean King, have used visualization techniques to improve physical performance. Michael Phelps, the most decorated Olympian to date, credits his success to visualization.

What's more, a survey conducted at the US Olympic Training Center in Colorado Springs revealed that 100 per cent of coaches and 97 per cent of athletes used imagery to enhance performance; 80 per cent of athletes reported applying visualizations to prepare for competition; 44 per cent practised it when learning new skills; and 40 per cent used it for relaxation.[21]

The effects of mental imagery are fascinating, as researchers outline that it helps to grow muscle strength, decrease

---

21 Mallett, R, "Imagery and Visualization: Strength and Conditioning for the Athletic Brain", *Believe Perform*, members.believeperform.com/imagery-and-visualization-strength-and-conditioning-for-the-athletic-brain/#:~:text=One%20 hundred%20percent%20of%20the,40%25%20used%20it%20for%20relaxation

anxiety, improve concentration and focus, and positively boost confidence.[22]

When gearing up for a tough event, we can all benefit from visualization. I practise it whenever entering my psychological dojo before tournaments. The technique I use involves picturing myself in the midst of a sports competition, whether it's just moments before or during a fight. I immerse myself in the emotional state, drawing in all the positive emotions and feelings I can muster. I imagine myself as strong, confident and self-assured. I create a version of myself that exudes calmness, groundedness and readiness for action. In my mind, I rehearse the moves I plan to execute with perfect timing and precision.

Using mental imagery can be an extremely useful tool to use in order to tap into your empowered warrior spirit, achieve calmness, cope with stress, and tackle your fears. When practised daily, it will positively boost your self-belief and confidence. It can be practised any time of the day. You can do it while waiting at the bus stop, or after an evening workout routine.

22 Post, P G, Wrisberg, C A, "A Phenomenological Investigation of Gymnasts' Lived Experience of Imagery", Sport Psychologist, vol. 26(1), 2012, pp. 98–121; Ungerleider, S, Golding, J M, "Mental Practice Among Olympic Athletes", Perceptual and Motor Skills, vol. 72(3), 1991, pp. 1007–17.

EXERCISE:
VISUALIZATION FOR INNER STRENGTH

Imagine a stressful situation that you might experience in the future. Perhaps it could be related to a difficult boss, a threatening work colleague, or a drunk customer. Think about the reasons why this scenario is important to you – does the situation threaten your boundaries, your personal safety or the safety of others around you? Make sure that you visualize this situation as if it is occurring in the present moment.

If you are practising for the first time, it may be helpful to find a safe and quiet place where you won't be interrupted. Calm your mind and tune into your breathing.

Picture the scenario unfolding in front of you, in as much detail as possible. Explore your emotional reactions to the situation in a positive light. Imagine you are in control, feeling powerful and alert. Evoke the feelings of boldness and confidence. Visualize your physical reactions: strong body language, a powerful stance and steady eye contact. Imagine what you are saying, and how you are saying it. If needed, imagine advancing into a physical intervention: what moves do you employ, how quickly, and with how much force?

As you observe a positive outcome to the situation (withdrawal, conflict being resolved), tap into the feelings associated with having achieved it. Ground yourself once more through steady breath work. Immerse yourself in the experience, embracing it psychologically and physically.

Take Aways

- Visualization is a practice used by many athletes and coaches. It involves imagining yourself in a specific scenario as if it was happening in the present moment.
- Visualization can be a valuable tool for coping with stress, managing your emotions, or preparing for an event. It can significantly boost confidence and self-belief.

Mastering Effective Communication

If we want to become effective communicators, it is crucial for our verbal and non-verbal signals to align. When we articulate a message, it's important that our body language reflects our intentions and the meaning we intend to convey. If we say "no" while displaying hesitant body language, It can distort the significance of the message and have the opposite effect of what we aim to accomplish. Imagine being in an important business meeting where you present a proposal, while your body language exudes shyness and intimidation. Even the most insightful words will not carry the same weight without a confident stance, good posture and positive gesticulation. To better understand this, we can observe how some of the world's most successful individuals interact with others through non-verbal communication. Take note of Oprah Winfrey's emotional connection through body language, the power poses used by Beyoncé, Steve Jobs' eye contact or Daniel Craig's poker face, and you'll grasp the tremendous power of body language when employed appropriately in a given context. This type of non-verbal messaging can build trust, establish authority, and convey assurance and certainty.

Effective communication is not a skill reserved only for confident individuals, but is something that can be developed and improved upon by anyone. If you think about it, verbal and non-verbal exchanges occur in our everyday lives: at home, at work and in social situations. From simple interactions with bank tellers or vendors, to participating in group discussions or friendly chit chats, we are constantly communicating.

The issue is that most of us aren't aware of our own voice and body language until we see ourselves from an observer's perspective. For example, if you've ever rehearsed a speech in front of a mirror or a video camera, you know how enlightening this practice can be. Once you closely examine the verbal and non-verbal messages, you may start identifying cues in your body and speech that may not come across as convincing. These cues can include avoiding eye contact, lowering your head, fidgeting, hunching your shoulders, or having a shaky tone of voice.

If you find yourself assuming a closed and contracted posture or sounding timid, you'll recognize how this conveys less power and assertiveness. By practising at home, with a colleague, or with a specialist coach, you can learn to present yourself more convincingly.

One way to practise is to rehearse a speech or conversation on your own, either in front of a mirror or by repeating the words to the point when they start to sound more convincing, smooth or natural. Another approach is to do some role play with a friend. If you're getting ready for an important meeting or an event where you'll be dealing with challenging individuals or a group, having a practice partner can boost your confidence and prepare you for a difficult performance or interaction. Repetition and constructive feedback can be invaluable for improving your performance.

Another effective way to improve your verbal and non-verbal communication is through self-taping. Those of you who have delved into the world of social media uploads can probably relate to this. You may recall the initial fear and uncertainty when first trying out public stories or live streams. However, with time and practice, these tasks become less intimidating and demanding, eventually resulting in a more confident presentation.

* * *

The more you practise and analyse all of the subtle verbal and non-verbal cues you are giving off, the more you'll notice how they intertwine to create a congruent picture of effective messaging.

To improve your communication skills even further, you can explore workshops specifically designed for this purpose. They provide you with the opportunity to learn from a coach, either one-to-one or in a group setting. There are plenty of public speaking courses out there, and if you can't find any in your local area, you should consider online platforms like MasterClass, BBC Maestro, or Coursera.

For children and young women, engaging in public speaking or theatre can be an excellent way to practise and develop communication skills. Encouraging young people to participate in workshops or events that enhance their verbal abilities can be incredibly empowering. Not only will it make them more effective communicators, but it will also build their confidence and resiliency. Additionally, from a self-protection perspective, it will equip them with the knowledge and skills necessary to assert themselves in situations of conflict and situations in which they have to protect their boundaries. Another example of verbal training that can engage females is role play, where it is possible to practise how you might respond in various scenarios. These types of sessions are often offered in self-defence classes, where women can develop their communication skills while being put under pressure of simulated conflict.

By actively investing in communication training and by fostering the development of speaking skills among young people, we can cultivate a stronger, more confident community that is better prepared to navigate various real-life situations, from casual exchanges with their peers to facing strangers in vulnerable contexts.

Take Aways

- Non-verbal communication is critical in moments that pertain to our safety. Therefore, it's essential that our non-verbal cues align with an assertive and confident verbal approach when establishing boundaries and conveying important information to others.
- Effective communication can be practised in everyday situations.
- There are specially designed courses and classes for mastering communication, such as public speaking, theatre, and assertiveness courses.
- To enhance your communication skills, practise in front of a mirror, engage in role plays with a friend or record yourself and watch the video back to analyse it.

EXERCISE: SELF-TAPE

Choose the setting and record yourself speaking to a camera. You can start with simple statements, or just read out a message before you engage in an improvised monologue.

When you're ready for a more challenging scenario, envision situations such as confronting your boss, calming down an aggressive customer, or negotiating a deal with a stakeholder – anything that would typically add an element of stress or discomfort to your regular emotional state.

When preparing yourself for self-taping and analysis (the post-recording feedback), consider the following:

- **Structure well.** Make sure that your speech is organized in a way that conveys the right message, with an introduction, a main topic and a conclusion if needed.
- **Have the end goal in mind.** Keep your focus on the end goal in order to avoid distraction or getting off topic.
- **Stay clear and concise.** Don't over-explain, and stick to the statements that carry the most importance. Avoid complicated words, unnecessary expressions, or adding too many details. Stay on track without going off on tangents.
- **Adapt your voice.** Notice how you're speaking, making sure that you're audible. Pay attention to the pitch of your voice and your intonation. Try to breathe evenly and avoid sighing. All these subtle changes in your voice can convey attitudes and emotions, such as anger, frustration, a sense of control, or steadiness.
- **Pace yourself.** Don't rush the process. Use pauses where necessary and the right timing to clearly convey your message. Certain statements may need to be uttered slowly, to bring about more emphasis. On certain occasions, take pauses to let the message sink in before moving on. This can give the listener the opportunity to reflect on and process the information.
- **Avoid filler words.** Notice if there are any interruptions, including words such as "um", "uh", "like", "you know", etc. If you need to gather your thoughts, use pauses, take a breath, or take a sip of water instead.
- **Mind your facial expressions.** What do they convey? Are you smiling, frowning or raising your eyebrows? All these cues can communicate your emotional state.
- **Watch your body language, including posture and gestures.** Are you crossing your arms? Are you standing tall or slouching over? These postures can indicate a lot, from assertiveness to passivity.

- **Keep eye contact.** Check to see if you're looking straight ahead, or if you avert your gaze. Sustained eye contact is likely to be associated with confidence and engagement, while avoiding eye contact usually conveys discomfort and intimidation.

EXERCISE:
7-DAY EYE CONTACT CHALLENGE

The objective of this exercise is to increase your comfort and confidence in maintaining eye contact with others. You can extend the duration of each practice step over several days to ensure that you can perform each task naturally and with ease before moving to the next one.

Day 1–2: Start by practising with family members, your partner or close friends. During conversations, attempt to maintain eye contact for a few seconds before looking away, keeping it as natural as possible.

Day 3–4: When you feel ready, extend your eye contact with your friends and family to more than five seconds. Pay attention to how you feel and if necessary, continue this step for a longer duration until you feel confident.

Day 5–6: Practise maintaining eye contact with acquaintances and colleagues during casual conversations, aiming for at least five seconds of eye contact. Try to maintain confidence in this approach.

Day 7: Once you have successfully completed days 5–6, challenge yourself by testing your eye contact with strangers. For example, try looking at a barista when ordering coffee or a vendor when buying groceries. Note the duration of your eye contact, and if you find yourself turning away in less than five seconds, continue this step for as many days as needed to be able to maintain eye contact for five seconds or longer.

While you try maintaining eye contact with friends and strangers alike, remember that this practice needs to be built gradually, and that breaking eye contact has to occur naturally from time to time.

It's important to note that in certain cultures making eye contact may be considered impolite, disrespectful or even aggressive. Make sure that you apply this practice exercise only in places where it is safe and reasonable to do so.

Power pose

Power pose is an open and expansive stance that often comes naturally to us when we experience significant life events, such as winning a competition, or receiving great news.

Our bodies instinctively respond, and adopt a strong and steady posture, making us look bigger as we take up more space.

The power pose, also referred to as "postural feedback effect" by author Amy Cuddy, is a pose that makes us feel more powerful. Amy Cuddy and her colleague's research at Harvard revealed that standing in a power pose for just two minutes increased confidence-associated hormones by 20 per cent and reduced cortisol (the stress hormone) by 25 per cent.[23] Subsequent studies have also confirmed that

23 Carny, D, Cuddy, A, Yap, A, "Review and Summary of Research on the Embodied Effects of Expansive (vs. Contractive) Nonverbal Displays", faculty.haas.berkeley.edu/dana_carney/pdf_Summary_Expansiveness.pdf

assuming expansive poses can enhance people's feelings of power and confidence.

I personally teach the power pose at various workshops as a means to prepare for potentially stressful and challenging situations. Assuming this particular stance even for a few seconds can contribute to a greater sense of control, and in terms of our safety, it can help us project strength and assurance. In this way, the implications are two-fold. Besides boosting confidence and competence, adopting a power pose also aids in emotional self-regulation and improved performance.

While power pose is not something you would use if someone approached you with an unknown, or potentially threatening intent (distance control and framing would be more appropriate here, which will be discussed in Chapter 4), assuming this pose as a way of preparation can be an invaluable confidence-boosting tool.

For years, I've used the power pose before important meetings (usually assuming the pose in a nearby bathroom) and in the minutes prior to competition matches (in the warm-up area). If you haven't tried it before, use the exercise below to test it, making note of how it makes you feel.

EXERCISE: ASSUMING THE POWER POSE

- Stand up straight with your feet apart, facing ahead.
- Place your palms on your hips.
- Project your chest forward and point your chin slightly up.
- Maintain a steady gaze.
- Stay in this position for least 30 seconds, up to two minutes.

Fake it Until You Make it

You may have heard the phrase "fake it until you make it" before. Whether you like to admit it or not, at one point in your life you probably employed a strategy where you intentionally acted or behaved in a way that appeared more confident than you actually felt in that moment. We've all been there, and as it turns out, this technique can be more helpful than most of us give it credit for. The underlying principle behind this so-called "faking" is to adopt behaviours and attitudes that may feel artificial or inauthentic at first, yet which can help us develop the qualities we aspire to possess. In moments when we feel insecure, projecting an image of a powerful self can influence how others perceive us. If, for example, we fake being strong and competent, people will see us in those ways. This in turn contributes to our own sense of inner confidence, which can be cultivated over time.

This technique, also referred to as "acting as if", was employed by Austrian psychiatrist and psychotherapist Alfred Adler as a therapeutic approach. Adler suggested that if one desires to acquire a certain quality of character, they should act as if they already possess it. By projecting an image of desired qualities and attitudes, this helps individuals to gradually shape their thoughts and feelings about their identity in positive ways, leading to increased self-confidence through consistent practice and internalization of those behaviours and experiences. The "acting as if" technique inadvertently influences our self-perception and can aid in adopting new patterns of thinking.

"Fake it until you make it" is another psychological tool that has also received validation from neuroscience. A similar method used today, often referred to as role play, can be employed in a similar manner, with the adoption of powerful postures and messaging.

Role play can be used in self-defence workshops, where we enact various characters to practise appropriate responses. We can do role play by assuming the roles of offenders, defenders, harassers, and those being harassed. This immersive experience incorporates facial expressions, body language and verbal responses to practise embodying the version of ourselves we aspire to become – strong, powerful and assertive. By acting and faking those new self-expressions, we can tap into our desired powerful female warrior spirit, one that is ready to face conflict, tackle aggressors, and ward off harassers, both in the role play environment and in real life.

EXERCISE: "FAKE IT UNTIL YOU MAKE IT" ROLE PLAY

In this role play exercise I would like you to work with a trusted person, someone who you feel comfortable and safe with. It could be a family member, a friend or a self-defence instructor. Here is how you can practise:

- Determine the scenario you want to work on. For example, imagine a situation in which a stranger comes into close proximity, taking up some of your personal space.
- Assign roles to each other – one person will act out the role of the aggressor, and the other person will act as the defender.
- Decide on the location and any props needed for this role play which may be helpful. The more immersive the experience, the more realistic it will feel.
- Begin with the aggressor moving in, as the other person asserts themself using the verbal and non-verbal techniques discussed earlier.

- Give each other feedback. Check for body language, eye contact, and assess the response by telling your partner how they can improve their reactions.
- Repeat this scenario as many times as you like so that it feels as natural as possible, gradually increasing your level of confidence.
- This role play practice can also advance into additional physical responses, which we will discuss in Chapter 5. These can be incorporated once we have reviewed the physical reactions such as distance control and framing.

I encourage all parents to use this role play with their kids, often reminding them of the power of communication and verbal responses, which they can employ when interacting with people they know, and with strangers.

Take Away

- Tools to boost confidence and affirm a strong body language include self-taping, maintaining eye contact, using power poses and techniques such as "fake it until you make it".

Imago Dialogue to Practise Connecting

While most situations in life will provide us with opportunities to practise communication and assertiveness, when it comes to conflict resolution, you may experience discomfort and hesitation. One of the more subtle ways to engage with strategies for de-escalation is through the practice of Imago Dialogue. This technique, originally designed by Dr Harville Hendrix and his wife, Dr Helen Hunt, while mostly used by couples, can also be helpful when communicating with people in general, especially during arguments and difficult or heated discussions. This practice allows us to connect more deeply with other people and promotes empathy and mutual understanding, which are the cornerstones of de-escalation.

The Imago Dialogue can help us bond with another person in a calm and peaceful way. It has the potential to build rapport, without resorting to extreme emotions. It will engage the pre-frontal cortex (the part of the brain that regulates thoughts, actions and emotions) to bring balance to the conversation.

When used regularly, the Imago Dialogue can lead us toward expert practice of the first stages of de-escalation: creating empathy and connection.

EXERCISE: IMAGO DIALOGUE

Whenever you find yourself in a conflicting situation with friends or family, use the following steps and take note of how quickly the emotional charge loses its power.

The Imago Dialogue is the interplay between one person who is talking and another person who is listening, and creating a non-judgemental and non-argumentative environment for this communication to take place. While people can take turns in this exchange, it is important to follow the three-step process as we, as the listener, actively gather information in order to fully acknowledge and empathize with the speaker, before moving on to expressing our own feelings, emotions and attitudes.

Three Steps of Imago Dialogue

Mirror. In this stage, we are the listener, and we should repeat back to the speaker what we've heard them say. This repetition can involve using the exact words, or paraphrasing. This stage doesn't include any analysis or critique. The goal is to be as accurate as possible in our words, without changing anything or adding interpretations to what the speaker said. This ensures that we understand the person, that they feel heard and it provides them with the opportunity to clarify or expand on what they've shared once we've repeated it back to them. Mirroring doesn't involve responding, it's the simple act of repetition to confirm that we've collected the right information.

Validate. If our interlocutor does not have anything to add, we can begin validating their message. In this stage, we can confirm that what we've heard makes sense for us, unless, of course, we need clarification. We can always ask for more information if needed, and this will show our speaker that we're trying hard to really understand them. We want them to feel that we are considering their viewpoint, and taking them seriously. What's important in this stage is to let the speaker know that we understand their perspective (even if we may not necessarily agree with them).

Empathize: This is the stage where we consider the other person's emotional state. We can show empathy for what they are going through with statements such as, "I can imagine how this must feel", "I understand this feels awful to you", and so on. This can be an opportunity to engage with the speaker, and verify if this is indeed how they are feeling. This will build a sense of connection and understanding, and the speaker will feel seen and heard.

* * *

Please note that the three stages described above should only be used during low-level conflict, and won't be applicable when facing a sexual predator or an attacker.

The Imago Dialogue is a very subtle way to communicate when the goal is to calm a situation down.

It's where we remain compassionate, at the same time upholding our boundaries. This technique doesn't have to put us in a vulnerable position. On the contrary: it allows us to avoid getting drawn into drama, giving space for a conversation to happen without trying to rush the process, or acting out on emotions. Even if it feels difficult during the verbal exchange, try not to take things personally, and always have the end goal in mind – building rapport, connecting and avoiding the escalation of conflict. You may be amazed at the results of this practice.

Once you've become skilled at connecting and resolving minor conflicts with your loved ones, you can also try handling more challenging interactions with strangers and acquaintances, such as coworkers, neighbours, or individuals outside your usual social circle.

Imago Dialogue and de-escalation can be great tools for calming a situation, but these tools are also good at preventing arguments from turning into physical altercations. Since Imago Dialogue can be applied both in personal and professional settings, think about the various occasions during which you could potentially practise these methods. For example, if you work in customer service, or retail, you are likely to have to deal with upset customers from time to time. Similarly, if you're a social worker, teacher or health care provider, you may need this skill to calm individuals in distress or to prevent harm. In these scenarios you'll need to be ready to offer options, communicating with the individual by asking open questions, and even negotiating. When opening the door for de-escalation, you want to be ready to turn the attention toward solutions, patiently moving the person from the state of agitation into a state of calm.

Take Aways

- The practice of Imago Dialogue can help us connect with people in a peaceful and empathetic way. It can be a great tool for de-escalation, where the goal is to calm a situation down.
- The techniques used in Imago Dialogue should only be applied in low-level conflict situations, where there is no threat present. The techniques won't be applicable when dealing with a sexual predator, harasser or an attacker.
- Once you've practised the forms of empathetic connecting through Imago Dialogue with friends and family, you can extend this practice to acquaintances and strangers.
- When using conflict resolution tactics, especially outside of your regular social circle, you'll need to be able to offer options, negotiate and turn the conversation toward solutions.

Building Physical Confidence

Martial Arts and Self-Defence

When dealing with situations that can result in physical harm, our capacity to cope will primarily be driven by past experiences, especially previous training. Our skillsets and understanding of our own strengths can have a bearing on our perception of the event itself. We can be confident in our abilities, or we can feel weak and vulnerable. We may be overwhelmed by extreme stress, or have the capacity to stay alert, yet present and mindful.

One of the best ways to prepare your body and mind is to put yourself in close physical contact with other people, under controlled pressure. This is where regular combat sports, martial arts and self-defence training can prove invaluable. This type of training enhances your physical capabilities, including strength, speed, reflexes and endurance, enabling you to recognize your potential and to perform under pressure. As you gradually increase the level of difficulty, pressure and speed over time, your resilience grows, allowing you to handle challenging situations, and building a higher threshold for discomfort. This is when your confidence rises, providing you with a sense of empowerment and self-assurance in your capabilities. It also equips you with the ability to withstand pressure in challenging situations, and alters your perception of confronting various scenarios – which can mentally prepare you to stay in control, reducing the likelihood of extreme trauma.

Many of my clients who are involved in fighting sports and self-defence training have reported feeling more empowered and better equipped to handle conflicts and stressful scenarios. They often perceive these situations as being less threatening than they were before their training. For some, this type of training may be their first experience of being in a vulnerable physical position, while for others, it's their first time engaging physically without experiencing shock or panic.

With all the physical and psychological tools at play, martial arts and self-defence training translate into a decreased chance of extreme traumatization, on most occasions. To discuss that very phenomenon, I liaised with a UK-based clinical psychologist, psychological therapist and martial artist, Rita Velikova. Rita has practised various martial arts, including the Korean traditional art of Taekkyon, and a relatively new system of self-defence called Hosinsul, in South Korea. She considers these systems to be incredibly valuable in terms of building both physical and psychological strengths.

I connected with Rita to discuss how various defensive systems could help women tap into their inner power and establish a strong psychological base for potential threats.

In our discussions, Rita shared about the unexpected physical attacks she has faced, and her reactions to these events. As Rita recalls, she was able to constructively cope with anxiety-provoking situations during these incidents, and didn't develop any extreme emotional responses during or after these experiences. These events also didn't lead to the development of symptoms of pathological conditions, such as post-traumatic stress disorder.

We agreed that self-defence and martial arts training experience is a great tool in preventing extreme stress reactions during times of physical abuse or attack, or when faced with other similar triggers.

This led us into a discussion about reactive mechanisms, which are formed through specific physical training. Through the diagram that follows, presented in figure 1, we have sum-marized our hypothesis on how these training programmes can contribute to a less catastrophic, and more realistic, interpretation of a stressful event, with more constructive behavioural responses to it. We juxtapose this with the cognitive interpretation and the possible emotional and behavioural consequences of a stressful event for people who do not have previous similar experience.

The diagram is derived from our past experiences, and is primarily based on personal situational observations, and Rita's years of professional work in the clinical field, where she treated patients who suffered from trauma. While the diagram incorporates certain elements of cognitive-behavioural explanatory models, it is not intended to represent a scientific paradigm on this topic.

Preventing Trauma Through Martial Arts/Self-Defence Training

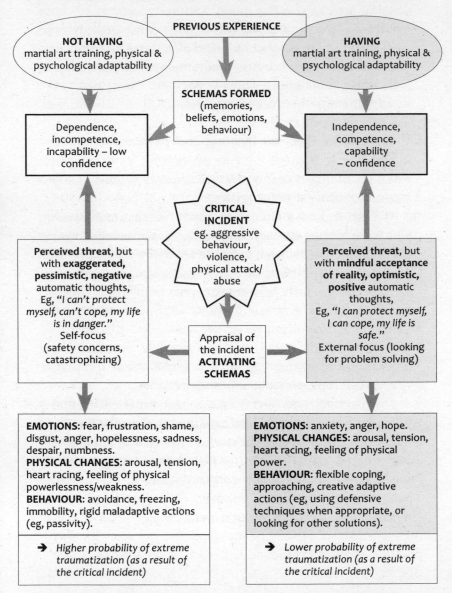

Figure 1. Preventing trauma through martial arts or self-defence training.

*The term "schema" mentioned in the diagram refers to the pattern of thought, a knowledge structure, which allows us to categorize, interpret and understand information. It's our framework of knowledge about the world around us, including people and events.

Take Away

• Regular martial arts and self-defence training provides us with the capacity to better deal with conflict in high-stress and anxiety-provoking situations. It can help generate more constructive behavioural responses, and aid in preventing extreme traumatization.

Other Forms of Physical Training

Various components of physical fitness can help you become a more empowered female. However, there is no one-size-fits-all format. Each of us should select activities that are relevant to our needs and those which we find engaging enough to maintain our interest, so that we keep coming back for more. Consider finding a training partner, as having someone to share the experience with will make it more enjoyable. Practising with a friend or a family member can also help you stay accountable and more likely to stick to your chosen activity.

It's best if the exercise routine you select is diverse enough to target different aspects of fitness. For example, if you're into weight lifting, you could consider adding in or alternating with some reflex work (in this way, you work both strength and speed). Similarly, if your main goal is building endurance, adding elements of either balance and coordination or flexibility and mobility could be an option.

Consider some of the following options for physical training, which will boost your levels of confidence, both mentally and physically. Recognize the benefits of each practice to understand how it can be helpful in a self-defence scenario.

Cardiovascular training
Cardiovascular training, or in other words, aerobic training, is a form of exercise that improves the cardiorespiratory

system, as it increases blood flow and blood volume to the heart. Typical cardiovascular exercises include jogging, brisk walking, cycling and swimming.

During self-defence workshops I demonstrate how the cardiovascular system works during reflex work in pairs. I schedule three 1-minute rounds of the game of tag, where partners aim to tag each other's shoulders. After this exercise everyone is out of breath, ready for the first water break. This cheeky little warm-up exercise is a demonstration of how quickly our bodies can become fatigued without previous training. Now imagine a scenario in which you need to get involved physically, but there is much more stress involved than in a game of tag, and the adrenaline is flooding into your bloodstream. The likelihood of you feeling exhausted in the first few seconds is quite high, and therefore conditioning your body for a better fitness response is going to be extremely beneficial.

To see results, you need to carry out cardiovascular activity ideally between three and five times a week, for at least 30 minutes at a time. If you can manage this, you will see noticeable improvements in how your body responds to situations when the heart is beating faster and more oxygen is needed in your bloodstream to continue to breathe.

HIIT training for endurance

High-intensity interval training (HIIT) is a training method that involves short, fast bursts of exercise with brief rest periods. In a HIIT session, you exert more energy than in typical aerobic exercise. Over time, your body adapts to the intensity, allowing you to handle other demanding tasks. Endurance training can greatly improve your stamina and turn you into a quick responder.

HIIT can be an excellent choice for conditioning your body to handle high-stress situations, especially when defending yourself. It helps your body react faster and significantly improves your ability to maintain your breath at a good rhythm. In situations where you need to run, your fitness level, speed and endurance will play a crucial role in your ability to escape the threat.

In order to see results in how your body conditions itself for high-intensity training, you ideally need to get involved with HIIT training two or three times per week, with 25 minutes spent on each workout. If you struggle to find time in your busy schedule, HIIT training can provide the perfect solution to condition the body, as it is the exercise option with the least amount of time spent on each workout.

Weight and strength training

Weight training is one of the best ways to increase strength and build muscle mass. The use of weights also boosts stamina and endurance. Strength training offers similar benefits, but apart from using machines and free weights, it can also include body weight exercises such as isometric exercises (static holds) and plyometrics, which involve using speed and force to build strength.

When getting involved in weight/strength training, consider consulting a fitness coach who can design a customized programme tailored to your specific needs and goals. If possible, invest in a longer-term personal training journey. In terms of consistency, aim for at least two resistance training sessions per week, ideally combined with other forms of exercise such as cardiovascular or HIIT training.

Weight and strength training are rewarding activities that strengthen the body in ways beyond physical force. They increase bone density and, from a self-defence perspective, enhance your ability to perform effectively under stress, allowing you to maintain stronger body frames for arms and legs, and to deliver more powerful strikes.

Other components of fitness

Other components of fitness that can contribute to you being able to move effectively and perform physically include:

Balance and coordination – this can be improved by the practice of yoga, Pilates, using body weight exercises, and free weights such as Bosu Ball (balance ball), TRX (suspension trainer), kettle bells or dumbbells.

Reflex/speed – this can be developed through martial arts, sprinting, plyometric training, and most sports that involve reaction time, such as basketball or volleyball.

Flexibility – this can be improved by stretching, practising yoga, and engaging in mobility work.

A great way to incorporate various elements of fitness, in addition to the previously mentioned martial arts and self-defence training, is by participating in team sports. Taking part in team sports not only enhances your physical abilities, but also fosters a sense of connection with others, adding a social aspect to training that makes it more enjoyable and motivating.

Take Aways

- Engaging in an exercise routine or training helps build physical and psychological strengths. Various aspects of fitness can be valuable for physical self-defence, including cardiovascular fitness, endurance, weight and strength training.
- Other components of fitness which can help in a threatening scenario are balance, coordination, reflexes and flexibility.

- For consistency in your exercise routine, it's important to choose a sport you enjoy, preferably with a workout partner who can provide motivation.
- An ideal routine addresses multiple aspects of fitness. Examples could include combining weight lifting with reflex work, or endurance training with balance and coordination.
- Team sports are a good mix of various components of fitness and add a social element to your training, which can increase your engagement and motivation.

Practice Charts

Given the various components of psychological and physical confidence discussed in this chapter, you have probably identified specific areas in which you can aim to improve your strengths – whether that's verbal or non-verbal communication, or physical fitness.

In the following Goals Tracker chart, please indicate the activities and challenges you're ready to take on over the next four weeks. For example, you may choose to start with practising mindfulness during the first week, then move on to the eye contact challenge in the second week. You may decide to get involved with martial arts training for the entire month and practise Imago Dialogue with family and friends during weeks three and four. Make sure your plan is realistic by selecting only the activities you can commit to within this timeframe.

Goals Tracker

MONTH AND YEAR:				
	WEEK 1	WEEK 2	WEEK 3	WEEK 4
MINDFULNESS & BREATHWORK				
PUBLIC SPEAKING				
POWER POSE				
SELF-TAPE				
EYE CONTACT CHALLENGE				
IMAGO DIALOGUE				
PHYSICAL PRACTICE				

After choosing your area(s) of improvement, it's time to track your progress using a habit tracker.

Habit Tracker

In the first column on the left, list the activities you have chosen to engage in. Track your progress by using a checkmark (✓) to indicate completion, or use a dash (–) to indicate non-completion under the corresponding day.

CULTIVATING CONFIDENCE

STARTING DATE:

ACTIVITY	MON	TUE	WED	THUR	FRI	SAT	SUN

ACTIVITY	MON	TUE	WED	THUR	FRI	SAT	SUN

ACTIVITY	MON	TUE	WED	THUR	FRI	SAT	SUN

ACTIVITY	MON	TUE	WED	THUR	FRI	SAT	SUN

Repeat this practice for as many months as you feel are required to improve your communication and physical strengths. Always keep track of the progress you have made.

You can download these charts from www.womenself defense.co.uk/post/she-fights-back-strength-charts. I recommend printing out the Habit Tracker and placing it on your fridge as a daily reminder to help you stay accountable.

Conclusion

A wide range of confidence-building tools are available for us to practise on a daily basis. These methods and exercises can enhance our communication skills, boost our self-esteem, and make us more self-assured in our physical skills.

In our pursuit of becoming confident women, it's essential to focus on developing a strong belief in our abilities. This foundation will empower us to effectively handle stressful situations when they arise. By engaging in various activities, such as public speaking and physical training, we empower ourselves to become stronger versions of who we already are, feeling more in control of our lives and more capable of taking action.

Take the time to carefully assess areas in your life where you can improve and enhance your skills. Create a roadmap to mastering confidence, and you'll enter a powerful realm of self-development, one in which the spirit of the female warrior is thriving.

CHAPTER 3
AWARENESS AND SPOTTING THE RED FLAGS

"Carefully observe oneself and one's situation, carefully observe others, and carefully observe one's environment."

—Jigoro Kano

One Saturday, coming back from her friend's house, Carol found herself at a busy subway station, waiting for her train to arrive. As she looked around, a man standing on the platform caught her attention. He blended in with the other commuters in terms of attire, but there was something about his demeanour that left Carol feeling uneasy. She couldn't quite put her finger on it, but there was an odd vibe about him. When the train pulled into the station, Carol observed the man getting on, and a strong gut feeling prompted her to hold back and wait for the next train. A few minutes later, she boarded another train, only to find it unexpectedly delayed. Shortly after, an announcement informed passengers of an incident further down the line.

When she finally reached her destination, Carol approached one of the subway staff to enquire about the delay, and learned that an individual matching the description of the man she had noticed had been apprehended for assaulting a passenger. It was a confirmation of sorts, reinforcing her gut feeling.

It's likely that you've found yourself in similar situations – where an unexpected event unfolded just as you had a hunch it might. We've all experienced this at one point or another, whether it's with acquaintances, family members, colleagues or strangers.

When I first started working in security, I was amazed at how accurately some of my colleagues could predict customer behaviour. I would often hear statements like, "This guy is going to be ejected within the next hour", and sure enough, minutes later, the same individual would be removed from the club. It both intrigued and fascinated me how brief interactions could lead to such spot-on predictions. Through my studies, I've come to believe that we all possess the ability to make accurate predictions in similar contexts, provided we pay attention and remain observant. By practising situational awareness and people reading, we can gain invaluable knowledge and hone our abilities to anticipate and avoid dangerous situations.

Situational awareness simply means paying attention to what is happening around you, especially when in a vulnerable context; for example, when walking solo in the dark. By being observant, you activate your inner compass, which will help guide you through various scenarios, as your intellectual and instinctive radars will be picking up cues from the environment.

In this chapter, we'll explore strategies for cultivating environmental and situational awareness, and strategies for recognizing predatory characteristics, modes of operating and manipulative tactics. We'll also focus on how we can employ proactive measures to ensure our wellbeing and safety.

The Nature of Violent Attacks

Types of Violent Attacks on Women

When we talk about violence against women, we're delving into a dark world where cruelty comes in many forms. Imagine moments that send shivers down your spine – a forceful slap, a hurtful push, a menacing threat that hangs in the air. These are the stark realities of physical violence that women endure, which sometimes leave visible scars, but which always leave invisible scars in the heart. Beyond this, there's also the chillingly wide spectrum of sexual violence – a reality we must confront. The terror of rape and attempted rape, and the invasion of personal boundaries through unwelcome touches.

We also need to remember that pain doesn't always take on a physical form. Psychological violence simmers beneath the surface, leaving lasting wounds that aren't always easy to spot. Imagine enduring insults, feeling belittled, and living under the constant threat of harm. This is the heart-wrenching landscape of emotional abuse. It can also transpire in short- or long-term harassment, where we may become controlled, living under surveillance, in constant fear of being followed or at risk of physical harm.

As we peel back the layers of violence to recognize when and how it manifests, we gain invaluable knowledge and the ability to incorporate certain safety measures. We become more attuned to our environments, and we empower ourselves to live our lives with more understanding than dread, more preparation than fear, and more confidence than uncertainty.

Stranger Versus Non-Stranger Violence

While perpetrators of violent crimes come from diverse backgrounds and situations, statistically they all have one thing in common: they likely won't be a stranger to their victims.

While muggings and random street harassment are usually crimes committed by people you have never met, sexual offenders and those responsible for more serious crimes are likely to be people we *have* interacted with in the past. This is a well-established fact, as acts of violence such as sexual assault and homicide are widely studied. These crimes, therefore, provide us with substantial statistical data. While these are some of the more extreme forms of victimization, the statistics shed light on who the most threatening offenders really are.

What we know is that women typically experience violent attacks from intimate partners, family members or acquaintances, which includes colleagues, neighbours and individuals connected through social circles.[24] Statistics reveal that violence against women, including physical and sexual assault, predominantly comes from intimate partners.[25]

Even in extreme cases like homicide, the statistics show that a majority of female victims are acquainted with the perpetrator. As an example, a 2020/2021 UK study revealed that in 54 per cent of female homicide cases, the suspect was a partner or ex-partner.[26] Studies conducted in the US present similar statistics, estimating that about three-quarters of all homicides involve non-strangers, with only one-quarter involving strangers. Intimate partners such as spouses, ex-spouses, current and former partners, as well as other

---

24 World Health Organization, "Global and Regional Estimates of Violence Against Women: Prevalence and Health Effects of Intimate Partner Violence and Non-Partner Sexual Violence", 2021, pp. 47–8, apps.who.int/iris/bitstream/handle/10665/85239/9789241564625_eng.pdf
25 US Department of Justice, "Prevalence, Incidence, and Consequences of Violence Against Women: Findings From the National Violence Against Women Survey", *National Institute of Justice Centers for Disease Control and Prevention*, 1998, www.ojp.gov/pdffiles/172837.pdf
26 UK Ministry of Justice, "Women and the Criminal Justice System 2021", *National statistics*, 2022, www.gov.uk/government/statistics/women-and-the-criminal-justice-system-2021/women-and-the-criminal-justice-system-2021

relatives, account for nearly 30 per cent of all homicides.[27] This aligns with a wider global statistic, which suggests that 38 per cent of all murders perpetrated against women have been committed by intimate partners.[28]

These statistics call for a deeper inquiry into the characteristics of both strangers and non-strangers who commit acts of violence against women. This will not only help you, the reader, to understand the statistical landscape of threats, but it will but also empower you, as an observer, to identify how women within your social sphere might be at risk and in need of assistance. By recognizing prevalent threats, we can begin the process of building a safer community where females feel valued, heard and protected.

* * *

Certain precautions can be implemented immediately. These include avoiding the over-consumption of alcohol, and never leaving your drinks unattended, as they can be spiked with drugs such as Rohypnol, ketamine or ecstasy. When slipped into a cup or a glass, these drugs are hard to detect and often will not change the colour or taste of the drink.

To show how alcohol consumption is linked to violence, consider the statistic which reveals that 55 per cent of female students involved in acquaintance rape were under the influence of either alcohol or drugs.[29] Influenced by these substances, one can lose motor control, memory, consciousness, and the ability to decide about consent. On

27 Messner, S F, Deane, G, & Beaulieu, M, "A Log-Multiplicative Association Model for Allocating Homicides with Unknown Victim-Offender Relationships", Criminology, vol. 40, 2002, pp. 457–79.
28 World Health Organization, "Global and Regional Estimates of Violence Against Women: Prevalence and Health Effects of Intimate Partner Violence and Non-Partner Sexual Violence", 2021, p. 31, apps.who.int/iris/bitstream/handle/10665/85239/9789241564625_eng.pdf
29 Rape and Domestic Violence Information Center, Inc (RDVIC), "National Statistics", info.rdvic.org/sexual-violence/national-statistics

top of that, combining alcohol with certain drugs can further destabilize our ability to cope and function.

With this being said, it is paramount to acknowledge that both stranger and non-stranger violence, such as sexual assault, is *never* the victims' fault. Irrespective of their attire, their whereabouts, and whether or not they were under the influence of alcohol or drugs, women should never be forced or coerced into acts against their will. While perpetrators of violent crimes always hold 100 per cent responsibility for their acts, we can try to protect ourselves by staying aware and present.

Spontaneous Versus Premeditated

Acts of violence against women can exhibit a range of diverse characteristics. Some acts are spontaneous and triggered by certain circumstances, while others are more premeditated, requiring a higher level of planning. Both spontaneous and premeditated actions may come from strangers and non-strangers, and will depend on the motives, emotional state, and the mode of operating of the individual involved.

Imagine first the spontaneous acts – those fuelled by intense emotions like anger, desperation, fear or frustration. These could include crimes such as mugging, street harassment, or sudden physical altercations like pushing, hitting or slapping. They can stem from things like a thirst for power, lack of impulse control, or feelings of entitlement and objectification. These impulsive actions might also involve sexual and psychological abuse, and often take place after heated arguments. During these instances, the perpetrator usually doesn't consider the consequences, as a rush of emotions drives their actions in the heat of the moment.

On the other hand, premeditated acts of violence are distinct in their calculated and intentional nature as compared to spontaneous or impulsive acts. They're typically carefully planned well in advance, and involve a deliberate intent to cause harm or injury. Sometimes, these acts begin with stalking, and escalate into something more sinister, such as abduction.

They can arise from motives like jealousy or a desire for control. Various complex factors often contribute to these premeditated attacks, including personal grievances, ideological beliefs, revenge, power dynamics or criminal intent. In the realm of sexual violence against women, premeditated acts often stem from deeply entrenched misogynistic attitudes, and are driven by a desire to dominate.

Although the calculated nature of premeditated attacks can be scary and unsettling to explore, it also provides us with the opportunity to familiarize ourselves with the discernible steps of their planning. This knowledge can help us predict and prevent violence before it takes root.

Take Aways

- Acts of violence can be spontaneous in nature, or premeditated and thought out with meticulous planning.
- Given the fact that a significant portion of violent acts against women are premeditated, understanding the steps leading to these attacks enables us to take proactive measures to prevent crime.

Premeditated Attacks

In preplanned criminal acts, predatory individuals usually follow certain steps to carry out their attacks. Their primary objective is to minimize the risk of detection. They may meticulously observe and then select vulnerable targets, employing tactics like grooming and manipulation to establish trust or gain compliance over time. Becoming familiar with these steps will help you gain a better understanding of how and when you may fall victim.

Observation and Assessment

In this phase, routines and everyday patterns might be monitored. Think of it as a study of where you go and what you do. Throughout this watch, even your physical presence and the way you carry yourself may be examined. The presence of those dear to you, or your social circle, might also be taken into consideration.

Identifying Opportunity

During this stage, the wrongdoer will aim to engage with the selected target. They will use the information gathered earlier to discern moments when the person might have less support or be without the presence of companions.

The Testing Phase, aka, the Interview

This phase is like a preliminary test before a potential threat, and is sometimes referred to as an "interview" stage. It's where boundaries are lightly prodded, and where a person's confidence and willingness are evaluated. It's a moment when choices are made, and someone might seek to separate you from your surroundings.

The testing phase can begin with a simple chat, as a way for the criminal to establish a connection to nudge you toward agreeing with their wishes. It could be as casual as asking for your number, or suggesting a ride in their car or that you join them in a hotel room. At first glance, this interview-like phase might not set off any warning bells. Those who test might use psychological strategies to disarm you, to lure you into a sense of compliance. Think of the criminal as being like a seasoned salesperson who can convince you to buy something you don't need – strategic predators can have a similar power to manipulate and to guide you toward actions you wouldn't typically consider. Their persuasion skills can be quite remarkable. Taking a closer look at these methods in the next section will help you become more attuned to these behaviours and will enhance your ability to recognize deceit.

Such knowledge and awareness will add an extra wavelength to your instinctive radar.

Testing Phase with Non-Strangers and Online Connections
Let's think about the phase where you're just getting to know someone, whether they're a familiar face or an online connection. Imagine a scenario where an acquaintance suggests meeting up in a cosy spot. It's important to remember that even though you might know them a little, treating them like a new friend is not the smartest move. The same goes for work buddies or folks from your social circle, including online connections.

Those long, late-night chats on platforms like Tinder might seem like heart-to-hearts, but they don't always reveal the whole truth. It's like someone putting on a fancy costume and playing a character. It may well be an elaborately fabricated impersonation story. Stay alert, as many predators use the internet to take advantage of others. They might start friendly interactions or build connections to see how much trust they can earn. It may be a test to see if you're willing to open up and share personal information. If you find yourself in a situation that feels unclear, or not trustworthy, keep your feet on solid ground. Take a step back and think about how much you really know about this person before diving in too deep and engaging more intimately. It's easy to lose yourself in an artificial world, revealing just a bit too much. Remember that any information which you share can be easily used against you.

Selecting a Location
Selecting a location is a critical element in a predator's sinister playbook. As they carefully choose their victims, gradually build trust, and skilfully manipulate their target to gain compliance, they also strategize the perfect setting. Initial contact could happen anywhere, in plain sight or behind closed doors, but for the predator to strike, isolation becomes imperative.

This calculated move serves two purposes: it minimizes the risk of detection and strips the victim of escape routes. The choice of location can depend on various factors, including the intention, and the relationship between the victim and the perpetrator. If the predator is familiar to you and has the opportunity to interact with you alone, access becomes distressingly easy. On the other hand, if you're a stranger to them, they're likely to employ manipulation and coercion, luring you unsuspectingly to their preferred location. If they decide not to use any of these isolation tactics, or if the tactics fail, they may go as far as gaining unauthorized access to your own sanctuary – your home.

Gaining Access to Your House – An example of an attacker's chosen location can be your home, and they may try to access your home without your consent. In this extreme case, an attacker's first concern would be to catch you in a moment of solitude. This might involve them keeping a watchful eye on you from a distance before they even consider any break-in. This observation could stretch over a period of time, as they can study your routines and habits to pinpoint the perfect moment for their potential intrusion. If you spot anything suspicious, such as someone following or watching you, ask work colleagues or friends to accompany you home, and prompt your neighbours to remain vigilant for unfamiliar individuals in the vicinity. Most importantly, keep your emergency numbers within reach.

If you suspect an intruder in the house, aim to run toward safety, such as leaving through the back door or a window. If these exit routes aren't available, find a safe room, ideally with a lock, and hide there. Once you've removed yourself from immediate danger, call emergency services, and provide your precise location. You can also use one of the smart phone safety apps which trigger sending an emergency response to your saved contacts, notifying them that you're in danger, and providing your location.

Apart from emergency calls and seeking refuge in a secure room, it's a good idea to have permitted or improvised protective weapons with you (for example, using an umbrella to jab with). You can use these in self-defence, according to the legal principles in your jurisdiction. Bear in mind that if the intruder is armed, direct confrontation can be risky. It may be safer to comply with their demands (such as giving away money or belongings) in order to avoid getting hurt. Depending on the context and the intentions of the intruder, it's best to act in accordance with your best judgement and intuition, using a level of force that is both necessary and reasonable, given the circumstances, to protect yourself and to avoid victimization. If you suspect sexually motivated intrusion, self-defence may be your ultimate weapon.

Take Aways

- Preplanned attacks happen in a few stages, including observation and assessment, a testing phase and isolating or gaining access.
- During the observation and assessment stage the attacker evaluates the vulnerability of their chosen target.
- In the testing/interview stage, the predatory individual uses manipulation tactics in order to isolate their victim.
- In order to gain access to your house, the attacker will usually conduct surveillance. Remaining vigilant of suspicious behaviour or stalkers will be key.
- In order to be realistic about your safety, treat acquaintances and internet connections as strangers when considering engaging with them in private, or sharing personal information.
- Report any odd or suspicious behaviour to your closest community.
- Ask work colleagues or friends to accompany you home when you feel unsafe.
- Have emergency contacts or smart phone safety apps

at hand in case a situation becomes more serious or escalates.

- If you suspect an intruder in your house, seek exit routes, or hide in a safe place, and call the police. Use self-defence and improvised weapons as is reasonable and necessary, depending on the context and circumstances you find yourself in.

Body Language in Victim Selection

If you've ever been to Italy, you'll understand this well – we communicate with our bodies. Body language stands as one of the most crucial tools in social communication, and it has significant implications when it comes to potentially becoming a target of assault. Numerous studies have identified consistent patterns in the way assailants select their victims.

The infamous serial killer Ted Bundy once remarked that you can identify a potential victim by how their head was positioned as they walked. While this might initially sound far-fetched, mounting evidence suggests a solid correlation between body language and victimization.[30]

In an intriguing study conducted by Grayson and Stein in 1981,[31] non-verbal cues in victim selection were examined. Setting up a video camera on a busy street in New York, researchers captured on film people walking in the same direction. This footage was later shown to 12 imprisoned criminals serving sentences for assaults on strangers. The inmates were tasked with selecting potential victims. Subsequent analysis measured various movement types

30 Brooks, N, Fritzon, K, Watt, B, "'You Can Tell a Victim by the Tilt of Her Head as She Walks': Psychopathic Personality and Social–Emotional Processing", *Psychiatry, Psychology and Law*, vol. 27(4), 2020, pp. 538–57
31 Grayson, B, Stein, M, "Attracting Assault – Victims' Nonverbal Cues", *Journal of Communication*, vol. 31, 1981, pp. 68–75

on the spectrum of physical athleticism and coordination. Results revealed that chosen victims displayed either unusually short or long stride lengths relative to their body weight, shifted their weight laterally instead of forward, and exhibited uncoordinated movement. These gestural hints for victim selection highlighted that the participating criminals possessed the ability to identify such traits.

Similar findings emerged from a 2020 study that explored the relationship between psychopathic personality and social and emotional processing.[32] A connection was observed between psychopathy scores and a heightened perception of vulnerability. If you're wondering whether this implies that psychopaths are inherently more intelligent than the rest of society, the answer is: not necessarily. The authors of the study suggested that this particular skill might come from the fact that psychopaths are more observant.

Another study, conducted at a high-security prison in Ontario, Canada, surveyed 47 inmates, and demonstrated a prediction of victimization amongst the studied group.[33] In this study, inmates were shown video footage of people and were asked to assess whether any of the individuals would likely be targeted as victims. Lo and behold, it was found that those who were identified as vulnerable targets did indeed have a history of victimization.

If this revelation fails to astonish, it should, at the very least, raise an eyebrow. It highlights the immense significance of our body language in relation to the potential of becoming a target for an assailant. The victim cues identified in these studies include walking style (slow pace, short strides, uncoordinated arm sway, restricted arm movement), lower

32 Durand, G, Rutten, B, Lobbestael, J, "Exploring the Relationship Between Cognitive Abilities and Adaptive Components of Psychopathic Traits", Sage Journals, 2023, doi.org/10.1177/21582440231173823
33 Book, A, Camilleri, J, Costello, K, "Psychopathy and Victim Selection: The Use of Gait as a Cue to Vulnerability", Journal of Interpersonal Violence, vol. 28(11), 2013

body weight, a perceived decrease in energy, and dragging of the feet. This uncovers a tendency for violent offenders to focus on women with poorer coordination and weaker physical fitness.

It's unsurprising that those who are physically less able might be at greater risk of assault, as they are more likely to appear frail and less capable of defending themselves. With all of this in mind, we can discover strategies for projecting confidence that can help us appear less vulnerable and thereby avoid becoming targets altogether.

Let's first consider walking. By adopting strong and slightly faster strides, we can appear more confident and purposeful. Enhancing your physical appearance can also work to your advantage. This includes maintaining an upright posture (avoid hunching), keeping a forward gaze, and taking straight, forward steps. It's worth noting that individuals who are more athletic and coordinated often naturally assume such a posture. Engaging in additional physical activities such as gym workouts or group sports can also greatly contribute to improved posture and balance.

Another integral facet of a confident and assertive posture involves establishing eye contact and exhibiting positive emotional expressions. Consider the image of someone walking with a sad and despondent demeanour, their head and gaze lowered. Their posture conveys a wealth of information about their mental state. To potential aggressors, these signals serve as indicators of the levels of individual's strength in that given moment.

Also unsurprisingly, when analysed in studies, women expressing either anger or happiness were perceived to have higher dominance, while those with sad expressions were perceived to have much less.[34] This is not to say that you should force a smile every time you're walking to ward off

---

34 Hareli, S, Shomrat, N, Hess, U, "Emotional Versus Neutral Expressions and Perceptions of Social Dominance and Submissiveness", *Emotion* (*Washington, D.C.*), vol. 9(3), 2009, pp. 378–84. doi:10.1037/a0015958

assailants. However, if you feel threatened, this could be a good time to act confidently, and to avoid expressing your sadness or tiredness. Lastly, if you want to look more confident, you can also adopt eye contact with an approaching stranger.

* * *

In bustling cities like New York and London, people are often more engrossed in their phones than in making eye contact with strangers. Regrettably, in many places this culture fosters a tendency to avoid looking at others. This behaviour seems to offer a sense of comfort. Yet when you visit countries like Italy or Portugal, where it's more common to engage in eye contact with strangers, you quickly notice that you are capable of reciprocating in the same way.

But what does eye contact mean for us in terms of safety? If we think about our almost soul-revealing body language, eye contact plays a big role in that. Eye contact can indicate that you are confident, aware and present, and that you pay attention to your surroundings. Those with malicious intentions might notice that you have spotted them, and may therefore choose not to approach you.

In some situations, however, avoiding eye contact can be helpful. This may include situations in which you're trying to blend in and become less noticeable – for example, to avoid having to engage with a stranger acting suspiciously on a bus. In certain forms of de-escalation, eye contact can also be limited in order to avoid agitating the aggressor.

If in doubt about whether using eye contact in a particular moment would be beneficial or not, ask yourself – is it safe? If the answer is yes (for example, the stranger already spotted you and interacted with you) then use eye contact to project unintimidated strength. If it isn't safe (for example, if you fear that eye contact might enrage someone, or make them spot you), use peripheral vision instead to stay aware of your surroundings, observing, and contemplating your options.

Take Aways

- Maintaining strong and confident body language is an important tool to prevent being targeted as a potential victim. This includes coordinated movements of legs and arms, faster strides and an upright posture.
- When threatened, affirm a strong facial expression to exude confidence.
- Maintaining eye contact with strangers can prove helpful when assessing threats, when observing the environment around you, and in projecting an image of strength and fearlessness. However, it should be limited when de-escalating, or when you are trying to remain unnoticed.

Identifying a Potential Attacker

According to security expert and author Gavin de Becker, predicting even the most unusual instances of violence typically isn't difficult. According to de Becker, "The Human violence we abhor and fear the most, that which we call 'random' and 'senseless' is neither. It always has purpose and meaning, to the perpetrator, at least."[35] There are often a series of signs that can serve as markers for identifying when an individual might become abusive or disruptive.

In this section, we'll explore both "primary red flags" that are evident and straightforward, as well as the more subtle warning signs that may require a bit more awareness and analysis on our part to detect. We'll uncover the shared characteristics of violent offenders, including strangers and non-strangers, to reveal what they statistically have in common.

---

35 de Becker, G, *The Gift of Fear*, Bloomsbury Publishing, 1997

You'll also get a glimpse into the intricate ways in which these offenders operate, and have a look at the manipulative tactics that they employ. Get ready for an eye-opening journey!

Primary Red Flags of Aggressive Behaviour and Violence

During my years in the security sector, I observed a few distinctive features shared by typical troublemakers and aggressors – those with a tendency to become spontaneously involved in disruptive behaviour. I refer to these features as primary red flags, as they are blatant, quite obvious and don't require deep psychological analysis to recognize. These characteristics can be observed both in strangers and non-strangers. However, it's essential to assess them from a wider situational perspective and the context in which they occur.

Spotting primary red flags doesn't have to propel us into immediate action. These signs can function as personal safety radars, keeping us alert and focused. They can help you remain observant, vigilant, and ready to respond promptly when needed – whether that means stepping back, de-escalating the situation, or holding your ground.

Primary Red Flags

Signs of Substance Abuse – There is a strong connection between substance abuse and violent behaviour. It can be observed in both strangers and non-strangers alike. When we notice an excessive or problematic consumption of alcohol, illegal drugs, or misuse of prescription medication, this can be a predictor of an altered state, which can contribute to an individual becoming disruptive or aggressive.

Intoxication should be taken into account together with other physical and behavioural cues such as such irritability, nervousness and signs of agitation. When linked together, these traits can become warning signs and predictors of violent behaviour, leading toward aggressive acts or physical altercations.

When studied amongst non-strangers, the frequency of intoxication was the most important predictor in intimate partner violence.[36] Therefore, if you're looking out for warning signs in your partner or someone you've recently started to date, observe their pattern of substance abuse over time. It may become your first red flag.

Signs of Aggression and Impulsivity – These traits are frequently observed in violent offenders, where individuals struggle to manage their impulses, frustration and anger. This pertains to both strangers and non-strangers, and in both instances can act as predictors of someone becoming violent. Even though acting out anger (for example, shouting) doesn't always translate into physical violence, dealing with an agitated stranger is a sure-fire way for a conflict scenario to escalate in front of our eyes. Noticing signs of anger, especially when coupled with substance use, should raise your eyebrow enough to ensure that you remain observant and wary. Think about how quickly the situation can turn around, and when paired with external motivations, lead to criminal activity. When you observe these traits in your intimate partner or someone that you know, frequency of these instances over time can also act as a radar and a warning sign that the individual has problems with self-control and may become abusive.

Certain physical indicators can help determine whether an individual is agitated, aggressive, or under the influence of substances. These may include:

- **Gaze:** Erratic eye movement, unusually large, or unusually small pupils
- **Hands:** Sweaty, shaky or exhibiting uncontrollable fidgeting

---

36 United Nations, "Guidelines for Producing Statistics on Violence against Women", *Economic & Social Affairs*, 2014, p. 35, unstats.un.org/unsd/gender/docs/guidelines_statistics_vaw.pdf

- **Tongue, lips and chin line:** Excessive movement
- **Body temperature:** Signs of high body temperature leading to changes in facial and bodily colouring, such as flaming cheeks and redness.
- **Perspiration:** Excessive perspiration, noticeable both visually and through smell
- **Head movements:** Sudden or uncoordinated movements
- **Body:** Uncoordinated stride, excessive movement or reduced mobility
- **Voice:** Incomprehensive, slurred, sloppy, mumbled or overly noisy and excessive.

Remember that while the above physical traits may indicate substance abuse and agitated states, by themselves they do not act as predictors of violence. In the next sections we will look at other factors and characteristics which can help us determine whether an individual will become abusive or threatening.

Take Aways

- The primary red flags include substance abuse, aggression and impulsivity. They are easy to spot and can be assessed together as behavioural and physical cues.
- Certain physical traits may be indicators that someone is agitated, or under the influence of substances. These include uncoordinated or untypical body movements, changes in speech and unusual body temperature.
- The listed indicators are not directly linked to violence. They can serve as cues which need to be evaluated in the wider context of the individual's motives and behaviour.

Characteristics of Non-stranger Violent Offenders

Typical offenders exhibit common characteristics that can help us in assessing and identifying potential risks. The following list of traits applies to individuals who may engage in planned or spontaneous actions. Some of these traits won't be apparent and may require a deeper understanding of the individual. When interacting with people in our social circles or personal lives, it's helpful to keep these traits in mind. They can serve as indicators of a higher propensity for aggressive behaviour, particularly in the context of men's behaviour toward women. Being aware of these traits can make a meaningful difference in promoting safety and understanding.

The Characteristics of Violent Offenders

History of Violence – Past instances of violent behaviour serve as strong indicators for the potential for future aggression. When dealing with someone who has been reported or accused of violent acts, be cautious and consider this factor. Monitor their behaviour closely and spend more time than usual observing them in various contexts before establishing trust.

As for individuals who have already exhibited aggressive tendencies, there's a strong likelihood that they will display more anger in the future, possibly leading to more disruptive behaviour that could jeopardize your safety. Any information, whether from friends or your own observations, should be taken seriously. A history of violent behaviour may involve actions such as physical assault, threats, harassment or bullying.

History of Abuse or Trauma – Individuals with a history of trauma and childhood abuse may be more prone to exhibit these traits in adulthood. Attempting to predict whether someone who has suffered from past victimization will become abusive is a complex task, as environmental factors and personal experiences must be taken into account. One thing that we should keep in mind is that certain risk factors can increase the likelihood that a person with a history of trauma may turn to violence. These risk factors include substance abuse and untreated mental health disorders.

Lack of Empathy – Violent offenders frequently display lack of empathy and show no remorse for their actions. Absence of empathy among people we know becomes obvious through their emotional responses to others' misfortunes. You may have noticed people who are self-centred, dismissive of the feelings of others, and who are unable to comprehend situations from another person's perspective. This can manifest in the form of insensitive remarks, lack of emotional response when witnessing the suffering of others, and a failure to offer emotional support.

Here again, it's important to note that not all individuals with low levels of empathy will become abusive. In order to identify this trait as a red flag, we must consider it in conjunction with other behavioural cues and pertinent indicators we possess about the individual – for example, antisocial traits, narcissistic (self-centred) focus, substance abuse or personality disorders. Other factors that can increase the likelihood of that individual becoming aggressive are the exertion of power and control, and the suppression of other people's autonomy.

Manipulative Behaviour – Violent offenders often use manipulation techniques to deceive others when pursuing their goals, which can manifest in various ways. In relationships, these behaviours become obvious when someone is influencing you or making you feel guilty in an attempt to gain control. For example, a partner might encourage you to stay at home rather than engaging with your circle of friends, justifying this as being an act of love.

Another common example is gaslighting, which involves making someone doubt their own beliefs and perception of reality, sometimes leading them to even question their sanity. Consider a situation where a deceitful boyfriend attempts to convince you that something you experienced or saw was a figment of your imagination. Even if you catch him in a lie, he will vehemently deny it, calling you crazy. Much like the plot of Patrick Hamilton's play – in which a manipulative husband intentionally dims the gas lights in the marital home and then denies any change – individuals can use psychological manipulation to instil doubt in your perceptions and memories.

At times, manipulators will also employ the silent treatment as a way to "punish" their targets, leaving them feeling anxious and desperate for attention. You can recognize this tactic when someone suddenly stops communicating with you after a disagreement, or a conflicting situation. They hang up their phone, or simply refuse to explain their silence. If you observe this type of behaviour over time, this may be an indication that an individual is employing a manipulation tactic in order to make you feel guilty, punish you, or make you feel anxious. It becomes a red flag.

Another tactic may involve emotional blackmail, where the manipulator threatens to take certain actions to coerce you into agreeing with their wishes. They may also link their love or approval to your compliance, creating a sense of conditional affection. For example, they might use statements like, "If you truly care, you'd do what I'm asking you to do." They may even threaten certain consequences if you don't comply. This tactic is often used with the aim of making you feel guilty, or responsible for their emotional wellbeing. Blackmailers are often adept at enacting the victim role, exploiting your empathy by feigning suffering to manipulate you into agreeing to their demands. In extreme cases, they might even resort to threatening self-harm or suicide to gain your attention, or to involve you in specific actions or behaviours.

Jealousy and Possessiveness – Excessive jealousy within relationships can indicate a potential inclination to isolate females from friends, family or support networks as a means of manipulation and control. It often begins with the perpetrator asking many questions about your whereabouts, your circle of friends and typical daily routines. The offender will usually try and influence your decisions regarding who you hang out with and how you spend your time. He will most likely become jealous of your closest connections, especially your male acquaintances. He may turn up in various places unannounced, or even search through your personal belongings, in an effort to monitor you and establish control.

Poor Mental Health – Certain personality disorders and other mental health issues can contribute to antisocial behaviour and violence against women. Spotting a personality disorder can be difficult, as only trained professionals can properly assess them. However, certain signs you can look out for include emotional instability, such as mood swings, and intense and consistent behavioural patterns that deviate from regular norms and expectations. These behavioural patterns may transpire in the form of disregarding your rights, lacking empathy, violating social rules and the use of manipulative tactics. Some disorders can also involve impulsivity and aggressiveness. With time, you may also notice that these individuals may have difficulty with social interactions and maintaining relationships, both personal and at work.

Preying on Vulnerability – Predators exploit weaknesses such as low self-esteem, emotional neediness, naivety and physical vulnerabilities. This is closely linked to their lack of empathy and manipulative behaviour. Those preying on vulnerability may not be easy to spot early on, as they usually conceal their intentions by acting compassionately and with understanding, usually offering help and support. Their seemingly genuine kindness can progressively turn into taking control over your emotions and decisions. Imagine, for example, a man approaching a woman who just suffered a painful break-up, offering unwavering support, only to turn into an obsessive pursuer weeks later. He may start isolating the person from their closest friends, become jealous, and use manipulation tactics as described earlier.

In the self-defence scenario, the attacker will also prey on vulnerability, recognizing emotionally or physically fragile individuals whom they will choose to approach. They may use convincing tactics to coerce or lure you into decisions you wouldn't normally consider, or actions you wouldn't usually take – for example, joining them by yourself in an isolated area.

High-Level Strategic Planning – Violent offenders often plan their attacks using a selection process to choose their targets, picking the location and methods in which they can isolate the person. Some of those planned stages have been detailed in one of the following sections: The Most Extreme Modes of Operating.

Extreme Views or Ideologies – Individuals with strong and extreme beliefs may resort to violence to advance their agendas, such as attempting to control or penalize women. These views can encompass misogyny (the belief that women are inferior to men), religious extremism, or domestic extremism that centres around male authority within the family. In such cases, women may become targets of physical or emotional abuse.

While not all the above characteristics apply to violent offenders, and not everyone exhibiting these traits will necessarily engage in violent acts, recognizing these traits serves as a crucial marker on our detective radar. Considering that a significant portion of violent acts are perpetrated by individuals we know, vigilantly observing these signs can act as our saving grace. Identifying specific behaviours early and being adept at recognizing manipulative tactics can mean the difference between interacting with a potentially assaultive individual, or safely removing ourselves from the situation altogether. The sooner we anticipate and spot unusual or threatening behaviour, the higher the chances are of avoiding victimization. Individuals who premeditate their crimes require time to gain our trust before striking; by identifying their tactics and comprehending their nature early on, we can effectively stop them in their tracks.

Take Aways

- Perpetrators of violent crimes against women tend to share some common characteristics, including lack of empathy, poor mental health, manipulative behaviour, jealousy and possessiveness, preying on vulnerability and high-level strategic planning.
- Being adept in reading those signs and behaviours can help us assess whether an individual may become abusive or aggressive.
- Stopping premeditated abusers in their tracks early is the best course of action to avoid risks and remove ourselves from potentially threatening situations.
- It's important to recognize that while the traits we have discussed are linked to violent offenders, not all individuals exhibiting those traits will turn abusive.

Characteristics of Stranger Violent Offenders

Gavin de Becker identifies several behavioural cues and methods that predatory individuals use to disarm or groom their victims. These manipulative tactics often go unnoticed as they are quite subtle and appear innocent at first glance.
These tactics can include:

Charm and Niceness
This pertains to an act of manipulation which will only be evident once presented in a specific context, rather than as a pure trait of character. This can be observed as a stranger

being overly nice without a particular reason, or when using a deceptive smile in order to influence and deceive the targeted woman.

Too Much Information
This can be noticed when an individual gives more details than a situation requires, in order to make his story believable. Just like a trained salesperson, the manipulator can flood you with a pile of information which may be difficult to process. The tactic is to make you feel overwhelmed and divert your attention from what is actually happening. When you're bombarded with details, it impacts your critical thinking and creates confusion, disrupting your intuitive radar and the ability to stay alert.

Discounting the Word No
Predators frequently dismiss the word no. If you decline an offer, they'll often persist or try to persuade you anyway, completely disregarding your boundaries and undermining your lack of consent. This behaviour demonstrates a lack of respect and can indicate a sense of entitlement from the person ignoring your wishes. They may believe that they have the right to influence, alter or control your decisions.

When a stranger disputes or disregards your rejection or declination, it's a significant red flag which you shouldn't ignore. When it's present in a vulnerable context, and you suspect manipulation, the best course of action is to remove yourself from the situation immediately.

Typecasting
In this manipulative tactic, the individual seeks to categorize you into a specific group you don't want to be associated with. For example, they may accuse you of being racist, rude or inconsiderate. This strategy is used to keep you engaged, allowing them to turn the situation to their advantage. Typically, the manipulator's objective is to draw you deeper into

the interaction, prompting you to contest their accusations and prove your innocence. Falling for this ploy can lead you down a rabbit hole in which you may find yourself fighting to validate your kindness and authenticity, while being assessed for gullibility and susceptibility to coercion.

Loan Sharking

The predator will perform favours for you, anticipating reciprocity. This can involve small actions, such as helping you with your groceries, holding the door, or offering you a drink. It may also involve bigger commitments, such as assisting you with tasks pertaining to your home, or more serious personal matters. Such forms of assistance and support may be a sign of a manipulative tactic aimed at making you feel that you need to give something back. The predator may try to compel you to reciprocate the favour by engaging you in activities you wouldn't normally consider or agree to.

When you suspect a manipulative tactic, or feel vulnerable being asked to do something in return, clearly set your boundaries and keep your feet on solid ground, reminding yourself that you don't owe them anything.

Forced Teaming

This occurs when an individual projects the idea of a shared purpose or experience, even when none truly exists. Its intention is to create a perception of common ground between individuals. This tactic is often unveiled through the use of the word "we", indicating a shared experience. Whether it's suitable to use this word or not greatly depends on the context of the situation. Such a personalized approach would not usually be appropriate when a single woman, in a vulnerable context, is in the presence of a stranger.

While rapport-building words may be used to create a sense of connection, "we", when used by strangers, can indicate manipulative tactics and hidden intentions. Keep an eye on that "shared experience".

Unsolicited Promises

A significant red flag arises when a predator makes promises not to harm you, or assures you that they are not like other "crazy" individuals. They may go to great lengths to persuade you that they are a trustworthy individual.

Think of your latest interaction with a stranger: has there been an instance where someone felt the need to reassure you that they wouldn't hurt or harm you? The likelihood of such an occurrence is quite slim, as most individuals don't need to rely on words to convince you. Instead, they demonstrate their trustworthiness through their actions and behaviour, making you feel comfortable and safe.

Flattery

This tactic is often used to manipulate your perceptions or actions, and it can involve giving you excessive compliments. By making you feel seen, valued and appreciated, the predator can distract you, making you less vigilant and potentially more likely to ignore red flags and warning signs.

Through flattery, the manipulator can build trust and connection. You may become more agreeable, more easily persuaded and more susceptible to their wishes. When flattery becomes a habit, it can create a sense of indebtedness, where, driven by a positive emotional boost, you feel like you owe someone a favour. Praise should never feel like something you need to reciprocate, especially when it is from a stranger. If you're being overly adored, or excessively flattered in an unnatural fashion, stay rational and don't let your emotions drive you – someone may be playing you.

Helplessness

Predatory individuals often feign vulnerability to elicit sympathy and persuade you to assist them. This can manifest in various ways, such as pretending to be emotionally or physically vulnerable, and encouraging you to demonstrate kindness and support by engaging with them. They may convince you to help them carry groceries to the parking lot, or simulate a need for help at their home, just to prompt you to visit them.

While helping those in need is one of the most genuine acts of nurturing female nature, we need to be conscious that predatory individuals can exploit kindness by faking injuries, pretending to require assistance, or making you believe that you need to visit them.

When presented with a scenario where you're asked to help someone, make sure that you do so in a non-vulnerable context. For example, involve someone else to assist you, or offer help in ways which don't include being alone with an unfamiliar individual.

* * *

When dealing with sexual offenders, you will witness these individuals perform some extremely skilful persuasion tactics like the ones mentioned previously. These offenders are proficient at employing strategies to disarm, influence and manipulate your decisions before you can even realize it. They demonstrate persistence and can easily sway you. It's crucial to avoid falling into their traps and to disengage whenever you find yourself in a situation where your wishes or boundaries are being disregarded or neglected.

Take Aways

- Predatory individuals employ specific behaviours and tactics to influence your decisions and manipulate your choices. Becoming familiar with these tactics can aid in recognizing acts of persuasion and coercion.
- Some manipulative tactics include using fake charm, flattery, discarding the word no and making unsolicited promises.
- If you identify persistence and manipulative tactics, it's important to be aware that you may be dealing with a sexual offender.

Stalker Characteristics and How to Tackle Harassment

I met one of my stalkers on a train platform, while getting off a busy London subway train. He approached me with politeness, extending an invitation for a date. Approximately a week later, we arranged to meet at a nearby bar. During the meeting, I observed some early warning signs – the man displayed intense emotions, and his drinks seemed to flow endlessly. It became clear that meeting him again was definitely not a good idea.

After declining his proposal for another meeting, I encountered significant resistance. This marked the onset of new warning signs: persistence, probing questions, a dismissal of the word no, and allegations of me being "rude" and "unkind", along with claims that I "didn't care". After blocking his number, condescending messages started pouring in from other accounts, packed with accusations in an attempt to make me feel guilty, all part of his efforts to draw me back into his web.

It wasn't until I delved into the research of anti-stalking strategies that I came to realize that my initial rejection had actually been an invitation – and you're about to find out why.

When dealing with someone who is overly eager to see you again, and you're not particularly enthusiastic about it, there's a single strategy that you should use – honesty. It doesn't have to entail impoliteness, nor does it call for excessive friendliness. The way you choose your words will have a lasting impact on what unfolds next. How you convey your desires for future interaction, or lack thereof, may be the deciding factor between someone persistently pursuing you and someone deciding to let it go.

Security expert Gavin de Becker suggests that when picking a rejection message, we mustn't say that we don't wish to be in a relationship *right now*. Instead, we should bluntly state that we don't wish to be in a relationship *with that particular individual*, if we want to stop the pursuer in his steps. Anything other than a crystal-clear message will be perceived as an act of confusion, opening doors for further probing. The moment we decline an offer from a persistent individual, there should be no more engagement or messaging from our side. Any post-rejection communication will simply contradict the initial statement, and begin a negotiation process.

There is also no need to provide explanations for your rejection. Avoid offering reasons why you're unwilling to engage with the individual – for example, coming up with excuses such as relocation (which, unfortunately, I used in the case mentioned earlier!). Providing reasons creates conditional rejections that aren't genuine refusals. In the eyes of the pursuer, they become challenges which he will be eager to address.

Another aspect to consider during such interactions is the social conventions that condition women to be polite and non-abrasive. Forget about being overly nice. Examples of statements that can be effective in the rejection process may include:

"I do not want to be in a relationship with you."

"No matter what you may have assumed till now, and no matter for what reason you assumed it, I have no romantic interest in you whatsoever. I am certain I never will. I expect that knowing this, you will put your attention elsewhere, which I understand, because that's what I indend to do."[37]

What I've also learned after dealing with multiple stalkers is the importance of reporting the situation early to all relevant parties, including friends, family, co-workers, or authorities if necessary. Gathering as much information as possible about the harasser will prove immensely valuable. It will help establish who they are, especially when they're present around your workplace or residence. The more

---

37 de Becker, D, *The Gift of Fear*, Bloomsbury Publishing, 1997

details you can share with those close to you, the greater the chance will be of others recognizing and confronting the individual when the need arises. Useful information can include the individual's physical attributes (height, build, eye and hair colour, clothing style, gait), how they talk, their accent, and any other relevant characteristics. An accurate description can significantly contribute to protecting yourself from unwanted interactions.

If the situation escalates and you're considering obtaining a restraining order, it's crucial to assess its potential effectiveness. Restraining orders obtained early, such as after the first instance of rejection, carry fewer risks compared to those acquired after months or years of stalking, according to de Becker. Once an individual has ignored the warnings and continued his pursuits, the restraining order is less likely to work. It will carry more risk, as the pursuer has involved himself emotionally, or maybe even introduced threats or hostile behaviour.

Take Aways

- Avoid negotiating with stalkers. Use clear and precise statements without providing reasons or excuses. After firmly declining, cease all future contact to prevent inadvertently initiating a negotiation process.
- Inform your social circle about the stalker. Provide as many details as possible. This serves as a protective measure and may deter future contact attempts by the harasser.
- Restraining orders are most effective when secured early. Their efficacy may diminish if pursued after persistent stalking and warnings.
- If threatened by a stalker, swiftly inform authorities and relevant parties. Taking prompt action is crucial to ensuring your safety.

The Most Extreme Modes of Operating

It's 1975, and a well-dressed man with meticulously coiffed hair approaches an 18-year-old Carol DaRonch at a shopping mall, introducing himself as a police officer. He informs the young lady that someone has attempted to break into her car. Upon inspecting her vehicle, Carol doesn't notice anything significant, yet she agrees to accompany the man to the police station. Her instincts alert her that something isn't quite right; she detects the smell of alcohol and observes that the man is driving an unusual car for a police officer. As they drive away, Carol realizes she is being abducted. Panic sets in, and the man handcuffs one of her hands. She fights fiercely and manages to escape.

Carol was one of the victims of the infamous serial killer Ted Bundy, who later confessed to the murder of 36 women, yet experts believe that the number of murders is closer to 100, if not more.

The charming-looking Ted Bundy often impersonated authority figures to intimidate and coerce his victims. Posing as a police officer and convincing women to accompany him to the police station was just one of his many tactics. He would also feign injuries to lure women to his car, wearing fake casts or using crutches and approaching targets for help, exploiting their kindness. His distinctive modus operandi was the way he selected and manipulated his victims. Modus operandi (from Latin), or MO for short, is another term for "mode of operating", referring to someone's habitual way of working. In criminal law, it denotes a method of operation or a distinctive pattern of criminal behaviour associated with a specific individual. MOs encompass the strategies criminals employ to make victims comply with their demands. As seen in Bundy's case, one of his tactics was assuming an authority figure role to gain access to women.

In certain situations, attackers hide behind fake identities. There are also cases where real law enforcement officers misuse their positions to trap victims. Just look back a few short years ago and you may recall the tragic case of Sarah Everard, who was strangled by a Metropolitan Police Officer in London in 2021. Unfortunately, this isn't a one-off case of authority being abused to commit crimes.

Take, for example, former Russian police officer Mikhail Popkov, who shockingly admitted to killing 78 women between 1992 and 2010. He lured victims using his uniform and patrol car.

Similarly, in the 1990s, the notorious American murderer David Middleton exploited his role as a police detective to abduct and assault women. After his parole, he even posed as a cable guy, using yet another disguise to gain access to victims whom he would then abduct, torture and kill.

* * *

While these cases are some of the more extreme examples of criminal intent, they also offer us a glimpse into how attackers operate, giving valuable insight into potential warning signs and some of the manipulative tactics employed by the most notorious violent offenders.

Environments

Places We Come Under Attack

Many of us hold onto the reassuring belief that the majority of unfortunate incidents occur in dimly lit, abandoned alleyways, far from the public eye. Of course, the risk is indeed higher in secluded areas, making you more vulnerable, particularly when you're alone. But don't be fooled into thinking that criminal activities only occur in remote and uninhabited places.

Muggers, for example, often target bustling areas such as streets and shopping malls in their quest for potential victims. Think back to your last shopping excursion, where you likely found yourself distracted by busy shop displays and chatting away with friends. In these moments, vigilance tends to wane. The issue lies In thls lapse, as it provides an opportunity for the mugger to strike. It's crucial to recognize that crowded spaces do not always translate into safer spaces. A seemingly comfortable place can quickly turn into a risk area, depending on the circumstances.

Similarly, while our homes may feel safe when fortified with alarm systems and surveillance cameras that instill a sense of safety, the introduction of a stranger's presence can instantaneously change the landscape.

For example, during my younger years when I was in my twenties, I frequently hosted house parties. Among these gatherings, one stands out to me vividly, as a friend's plus-one guest created quite a commotion with his inappropriate behaviour. At a certain point during the party, he discreetly disappeared into the bathroom, only to reappear inexplicably draped in a towel after undressing. Swiftly and unnoticed, he ascended the stairs to the upper floor, where he proceeded to knock insistently on my flatmate's door, demanding entry. Thankfully, her startled screams prompted immediate intervention, as a group of jiu-jitsu practitioners present in the house swiftly stepped forward to restrain and escort the disruptive joker out. Similar scenarios can play out during other social events or public gatherings, where we may drop our guard and face a potentially dangerous situation.

While we may come under attack in every space imagined, statistical data on threats against women often include the following places:

Mostly Non-Stranger Violence

Domestic space: A large portion of threats against women occur in the form of domestic violence or partner abuse, which often takes place at home.

Workplace: Office buildings, factories and other places of work are some of the locations where harassment and abuse can occur.

Educational institutions: Schools and colleges are one of the most common spaces for acts of bullying and harassment, where assault and abuse can take place.

Mostly Stranger Violence

Public spaces: Streets, parks and public transport are common spaces where harassment and assaults take place.

Social and recreational establishments: Bars, clubs, and other entertainment venues are spaces where many unwanted advances take place.

Violence against women can happen in many different settings, across all socioeconomic and demographic backgrounds, and will depend on the type of criminal act being committed. For example, numerous studies conducted in western countries have revealed the significant prevalence of sexual assaults on women within college and university environments. Typically, these acts are perpetrated by individuals acquainted with the victim. Conversely, muggings might transpire in alleys, parks, residential zones and commercial centres.

We need to adopt a broader perspective to identify areas that present potential risks to our safety – for example, by linking this information with previously examined characteristics of predatory individuals. By assessing the space and context of the situation, we can become adept at reading the environment, and the people within it.

Take Aways

- Violence can occur in different locations, and varies based on the nature of the acts being committed. For example, sexual assaults are more likely to happen in isolated spaces, whereas muggings might take place in busy areas.
- Common locations for violent attacks include domestic and public settings, workplaces, educational institutions, as well as social and entertainment establishments.
- In order to become adept at recognizing threats, we need to observe both the environment, and the people within it, to spot where we may become vulnerable.

Environmental Awareness

It's clear that observing our surroundings can significantly heighten our awareness and readiness to respond to potential threats. This being said, maintaining a constant state of hyper-alertness as if our lives were perpetually in danger can be counterproductive and extremely exhausting. Scanning our environment doesn't have to entail relentless scrutiny or constant hyper-vigilance. In fact, over-alertness can undermine our survival instincts, as it directs our focus toward anticipated threats rather than actual occurrences.

Excessive sensitivity may lead us to fixate on non-threatening elements, distorting our attention. This fixation could actually make us overlook potentially menacing situations that demand our awareness.

In the course of our daily lives, our attention should be attuned to the contexts in which threats may manifest, and we should raise our vigilance as needed based on the circumstances. These potentially risky situations could include times when we're alone, when we're in an environment that doesn't feel secure, or when we're around someone who raises concerns.

Let's explore some scenarios in which our safety could be compromised – when it is therefore crucial to exercise caution and heightened awareness:

Unusual Behaviour of Individuals
Anyone who appears out of place or who triggers a strong gut feeling should be closely observed. Pay attention to body language and the behaviours outlined earlier as primary red flags, and remain vigilant in assessing the situation.

Poor Lighting
Diminished visibility makes it harder to assess environmental threats. In those moments, you can take extra precautions – for example, by opting for the better-lit side of the street, or by getting a taxi, especially when you find yourself in an unfamiliar area.

Vulnerable Times of the Day
Depending on the time, spaces can become more threatening due to decreased visibility and fewer witnesses. Any deserted space could potentially mean that you are in a more vulnerable situation. Paying extra attention in those moments will matter – listen, watch and observe your surroundings.

Threatening Spaces
Dead-end locations or confined spaces where mobility is limited can pose a risk to your safety. Try to choose open spaces when walking by yourself. Especially when in a deserted area, or when it is dark, try to stay away from corners, where potential attackers may be hiding.

Isolation
Being alone with someone unfamiliar can be threatening. If possible, avoid such situations altogether. If you decide to stay one-on-one with a stranger, it's a good idea to inform others of your whereabouts and who you are with. You can

request periodic check-ins from your friends or family for added safety.

Unknown Territory

Unfamiliar areas pose increased challenges in terms of recognizing threats, knowing escape routes, and being able to confidently navigate yourself. Exercising caution will be key, and this can include calling a taxi, having someone accompany you, or, if you're left with no other choice than to walk the route by yourself, staying more alert than normal.

Limited Communication

In isolated areas with restricted communication access, losing reception could hinder your ability to call for help. If you're invited by a stranger to a place with limited internet access, consider this risk to your safety.

* * *

The key in all of these instances is to pay attention to the surroundings while assessing your vulnerability. To hone your environmental awareness, you can practise observational skills in different locations, at various times of the day and night. You can use the following exercise to check how quickly you're capable of assessing your environment. The drills described in the exercise have been adopted from *Self-Defense: Steps to Success* by Joan Nelson.[38]

---

38 Nelson, J M, *Self-Defense: Steps to Success*, Leisure Press, 1991

EXERCISE:
ENVIRONMENT ASSESSMENT DRILL

Pick between five and ten locations that you normally visit during the day in which to conduct the assessment. These can be office spaces, social spots, parking lots, or even rooms in your household. Once you find yourself at each location, give yourself about five to ten seconds to determine the following:

- Escape routes and exits
- Potential hiding spots
- Barriers and shields
- Availability of improvised weapons
- Unusual behaviour of individuals
- Proximity of other people around you.

If possible, assess these locations both during the day and during the night, to identify any variations in the level of safety they provide depending on time of day. Take note of the lighting, weather conditions, and the level of crowding in these areas at different times. Also, observe the objects available around you. You can also try to spot any CCTV cameras that may be present, as this could potentially add an extra layer of security. Conversely, lack of cameras may increase the chances of harassers and attackers operating in the area.

Once you've conducted your research, you can apply this method for environmental assessment every time you enter a new space. You can do it when visiting a new nightclub, an unfamiliar neighbourhood, a new office space or a friend's house. The more you practise doing these assessments, the more natural they will become, ultimately forming a new habit.

EXERCISE: IDENTIFYING RISKS

In this exercise, assess the areas in your life where you can minimize the potential risk of being targeted by an assailant. Describe briefly how you can implement new safety measures, which can include avoiding certain places, or avoiding certain individuals, etc.

Take into account the following settings:

On the street:

*

*

*

At home:

*

*

*

At work:

*

*

*

In your car or on public transport:

-

-

-

In social spaces such as bars, restaurants and clubs:

-

-

-

Online:

-

-

-

By identifying areas where you can reduce your vulner-abilities and put safety measures in place, you can equip yourself with the know-how and tactics to boost your personal safety. Taking this proactive approach can help protect you and give you a stronger sense of confidence.

Cultural Differences

Life's a never-ending voyage of learning, whether we're living our own stories or watching from the sidelines. It gets even more interesting when we come across diverse cultures during travel, or when living in a multicultural environment. Exploring various cultures exposes us to situations which may surprise us, but also those that can get us into trouble ...

Have you even been in a situation where you showed affection when it was prohibited, or reached out your left hand for a handshake in a culture where that is considered impolite? Perhaps you have unintentionally worn clothes that were deemed inappropriate for the occasion, inviting disapproving looks?

Navigating foreign cultures as a woman can leave us vulnerable, potentially exposing us to unwanted attention, harassment, impertinent comments or even physical assault.

Consider, for example, the public display of affection in certain societies where this behaviour is deemed inappropriate. Such behaviour might be perceived as disrespectful and provocative, leading to tensions and escalating to verbal confrontations or even violence.

When you interact with different cultures or go on an adventure to explore unfamiliar destinations, remember to exercise caution. This will help prevent unintentional breaches of local customs. Some of these potential violations that you should be aware of include:

- Staring or maintaining prolonged eye contact
- Inappropriate or immodest dress code
- Invading personal space by standing too close
- Public displays of affection
- Interrupting ongoing conversations
- Taking photographs of locals without their consent
- Public intoxication or substance use
- Expressing political views overtly

- Mocking local customs
- Raising your voice inappropriately
- Ignoring gender segregation norms
- Engaging in politically charged discussions
- Displaying aggressive or disruptive behaviour
- Failing to remove shoes when required
- Using hand gestures that are considered impolite
- Carrying illegal items.

When planning your travels, make sure to explore social norms and customs through research (in books or online), or by getting in touch with residents who can teach you about local traditions and expectations.

Take Aways

- Social customs, traditions and norms differ across cultures.
- Disregarding these customs can result in unwanted confrontations and, in extreme cases, violence.
- Instances of breaching local customs might involve wearing immodest clothing, displaying affection in public spaces, or expressing political views overtly.
- When venturing into unfamiliar environments, it's essential to dedicate time to familiarizing yourself with the local customs. Doing so can help safeguard against potential victimization.

Intuition and Gut Feeling as Threat Detectors

During my refresher driving lessons, I asked my instructor how I could better anticipate the actions of fellow drivers. He told me to pay attention to the "body language" of the cars around me. Initially, I found this guidance somewhat confusing, and struggled to fully grasp the underlying concept. It wasn't until several months later that my brain had amassed enough practice behind the wheel to effectively decode the behaviour of other drivers – whether or not they would permit me to change lanes, or yield at intersections.

Much like this process, our brains continuously accumulate an array of information, enabling us to pre-emptively react to our surroundings in order to shield ourselves from potential hazards.

These pieces of information are often referred to as System 1, as defined by Daniel Kahneman, a Nobel laureate and author of ground-breaking work on human thinking. In his book *Thinking, Fast and Slow*,[39] Kahneman introduces the concept of two thinking systems that assist humans in processing information and making decisions.

System 1 is described as the intuitive, automatic system of fast thinking. It operates quickly and effortlessly, processing information based on patterns and associations from past experiences. This system enables rapid judgements and triggers immediate emotional responses. It stands in contrast to System 2, which is the slower, more analytical, and deliberate type of thinking that involves conscious reasoning and logical deduction for problem solving.

Therefore, intuition arises when the brain relies on past experiences and external cues when making decisions at a subconscious level. It often manifests as a hunch, an understanding without conscious reasoning. Intuition can take the form of a visceral feeling about a situation and may be accompanied by physical sensations in the stomach area, commonly known as "gut feelings".

Judith Orloff, assistant clinical professor of psychiatry at UCLA and author of *Guide to Intuitive Healing: 5 Steps to Physical, Emotional, and Sexual Wellness*,[40] explains that, much like the human brain, neurotransmitters in our gut

---

39 Kahneman, D, *Thinking, Fast and Slow*, Farrar, Straus and Giroux, 2013
40 Orloff, J, *Guide to Intuitive Healing: 5 Steps to Physical, Emotional, and Sexual Wellness*, Harmony, 2001

are equipped to respond to stimuli from the environment. When activated, they may produce a tingling sensation or discomfort in the stomach.

Researchers suggest that gut instinct plays a substantial role in our intuition. Often regarded as our "second brain", the enteric nervous system shares characteristics with the brain and can function autonomously or in conjunction with it. It communicates messages directly to the brain through the vagus nerve, exerting an influence on our behaviour. Operating beneath our conscious awareness, this enteric nervous system (which can regulate gastrointestinal behaviour independently of the central nervous system) assists in detecting environmental threats and shaping our responses to them.

Gut feeling or intuition in general can play a pivotal role in determining whether to disengage from a situation. It can aid us in avoiding potentially hazardous circumstances. When you experience it, be sure to validate it without trying to rationalize it. Use it to make decisions about your actions in the present, as these feelings can serve as strong indicators of potential imminent danger.

Aside from the gut sensation (tingling or discomfort in the stomach area), feelings associated with intuition may include:

- **Unease and discomfort:** A sense that something is not quite right.
- **Nagging feelings:** The sensation that something is off.
- **Strong rejection or repulsion:** Feeling strongly repulsed by a particular individual.
- **Dread:** A sense of impending danger, a feeling that something bad is about to happen.
- **Anxiety:** This can manifest itself as an increased heart rate, rapid breathing, sweating, nervousness, restlessness and irritability.
- **Curiosity:** Curiosity often accompanies heightened awareness and focused attention.

- **Suspicion:** Perceived as increased awareness and alertness, with a feeling of questioning or doubt.
- **Fear:** A primal instinct, guiding us to treat the situation seriously and prioritize our safety.

Our intuitive powers are remarkably accurate, enabling us to predict phone calls from distant friends, navigate traffic with precision, and even sense the gaze of someone upon us when we're not looking at them. Every second, our bodies provide us with a myriad of signals, helping us to survive and guiding us as we navigate through an ever-changing environment. In each moment, our brains analyse thousands of subtle cues across all sensory levels, offering insights into the external world. When we choose to switch off our robotic autopilot and observe intently, we uncover more than the naked eye can see.

Take Aways

- Intuition proves to be an immensely important tool for predicting potentially threatening situations.
- A pivotal aspect of intuition is the visceral feeling that is often experienced in the gut area.
- Additional forms of intuitive feelings may encompass unease, discomfort, anxiety, suspicion, strong repulsion, dread and fear.

Conclusion

The more we learn about violent attacks, the more it becomes evident that we need to understand the distinct and unique traits exhibited by those who commit acts of violence against women. By analysing predatory characteristics and behaviours, we equip ourselves with a discerning eye for red flags, warning signs and pre-attack indicators. Armed with this awareness, we can empower ourselves to effectively counter approaches by potential aggressors.

It's also crucial to understand where violent attacks might happen – both in familiar places (with strangers and non-strangers alike), as well as in unfamiliar territories. By keeping an eye on our surroundings and addressing vulnerable situations and stalking cases early, we boost our personal safety and mitigate risks across a spectrum of encounters. With this knowledge and some proactive steps under our belt, we can become more confident as we navigate various situations in our personal and professional lives.

In addition, using intuition as our safety radar can help us in identifying potential threats, as it serves as a warning sign and a protective measure. Gut feelings associated with intuition can act as our inner guidance system, informing us of a potentially hazardous situation. Staying attuned to this intuitive radar can be crucial in safeguarding our wellbeing.

CHAPTER 4
FACING CONFLICT

"Move swift as the Wind and closely-formed as the Wood. Attack like the Fire and be still as the Mountain."

—Sun Tzu

A few years ago, on a summer afternoon, I was casually strolling toward Kilburn High Road in West London, when I caught a glimpse of someone moving behind me. The area appeared calm and mostly empty, so I decided to take a precautionary measure and cross the street. Within seconds, I noticed the man synchronizing his steps with mine and closing the distance between us. I decided to stop and address him face to face. I turned around and fired a couple of questions, just to witness his sly grin transform into a neutral expression as he walked away.

What happened for me in that situation could have been very different for someone else. Some might have chosen to run, or to shout out for help, which may have been the right move for them in that given moment. We should always assess each situation individually, considering the level of threat present, our skills, confidence, and our intellectual and physical reactions.

My decision in that scenario was mainly based on strategies and behaviours I'd learned over time. They involved listening to the inner voice of my intuition, checking for escape routes, using peripheral vision to assess the stranger's build and demeanour, and drawing on my previous training experience. All of these tools are crucial when making quick decisions in moments of perceived danger.

* * *

Have you ever found yourself in a situation where you confronted someone, and noticed several determining factors at play, possibly influenced by your past experiences? Some of these reactions may have been instinctual, while others may have been made on a rational level. Reassuringly, both types of response can be cultivated over time, enabling you to gain a better understanding of how to prepare yourself for an even more effective response in later stressful scenarios.

In this chapter we will explore the different stages of conflict, including assessment, different psychological and linguistic techniques you can use, and how to retreat to safety. We will discuss the physiological changes our bodies undergo during high-stress situations, in order to understand how this may impact your reactions and performance. We will also introduce a strategy for calming your nervous system during such scenarios.

Mindful Assessment

Let's envision a scenario where you find yourself faced with an unsettling or potentially dangerous situation – a sudden encounter with someone on a secluded pathway, catching you off guard. Your capacity to stay alert to what is happening around you will be pivotal in determining your response. Remaining present while under stress will impact the way you react and behave. Being mindful will also mean acknowledging your strengths, your abilities, and your current mental state. It will enable you to stay alert yet composed, sustaining focus without losing your way, and it will allow you to stay realistic about your circumstances. You will act based on the knowledge and awareness of your skills and strengths, and you will be able to objectively strategize, swiftly and deliberately taking steps to ensure your safety.

To illustrate mindfulness assessment at play, I often share a story from my teenage years, when I was assaulted by a stranger. This incident occurred when I was about 16 years old, as I was leisurely strolling in a forest on a summer afternoon. As I walked, admiring the wildlife, I suddenly felt someone's hand on my shoulder, forcefully pulling my jacket from behind. Emerging from the bushes was a man, stark naked except for his underwear briefs which were placed on top of his head. My body reacted with a sudden jolt as fear coursed through me, catching me a bit off guard. I shouted out for help, while trying to free myself from the man's grip. I started throwing kicks at his body, pressuring him to let go. When I was ready to retreat, the stranger seized my bag. At that moment, I faced two choices: surrender my belongings and run, or continue fighting. Determined not to give up, I kept screaming and kicking, while the man remained still, without any intention of letting go or retaliating. He remained motionless, observing my reactions. Eventually, I gave in and ran off, filled with regret for leaving my backpack behind, but relieved that the stranger didn't follow me.

Was it dangerous of me to stay and fight in that moment? How did I know the man wouldn't drag me into the bushes, or overpower me? I realized later that what guided my reactions was my ability to assess the risk, and to objectively analyse the facts in the moment, without being consumed by emotions. I most likely determined the level of threat before deciding on my actions. In a fraction of a second, I had the opportunity to examine the man's appearance (weight, height, build) and his gaze, which allowed me to make an informed decision on how to proceed.

The next factor that contributed to my decision to fight was my kickboxing background and my physical capabilities, which played a subconscious role in my response. In that moment, my mind was infused with strong self-talk, affirming that I was able to handle the situation. I also reacted militantly, issuing various verbal demands for the man to let go, as my body acted on reflexes honed from hours of training in the martial arts dojo. As I threw the first kick, it became evident that the man had no intention of fighting back. His stance and appearance indicated his unwillingness to engage in a physical exchange. Upon reflecting on the event, it became clear that the mysterious man who attacked me from the bushes was an exhibitionist, deriving sexual pleasure from exposing himself naked. There were multiple signs that suggested he was not a typical sexual predator, but rather a mentally disturbed individual. His lack of attire, static posture, gaze filled with excitement, and limited physical activity, all indicated that he was not going to harm me.

In the moment of unprecedented shock, staying mindful, calm and attentive was what drove my decisions and saved me from freezing. In the same way, your initial assessment will be crucial in such scenarios. In the first instance, you will want to ask yourself whether there is a way out of the situation without resorting to physical violence. Are there any escape routes? Can you run toward safety, and if so, where to? Are you ready to de-escalate, or perhaps use assertiveness, and focus on avoiding physical contact?

These are all pertinent questions to consider when dealing with a potential attacker. By addressing them honestly, we can establish our competence and determine how best to respond. When facing the unexpected, the ability to remain calm, alert and present will be paramount in finding answers to these questions, and in taking effective action.

* * *

Picture yourself alone, with an unexpected stranger approaching at high speed with aggressive body language,
staring right at you. Do you freeze, speak up, feign ignorance,
or flee? If you have spotted this person early on, you may have
acquired enough information to consider your options before
acting. Perhaps a few seconds was just enough to trigger your
intuitive radar, or raise some red flags and determine that
you're dealing with a predatory individual who is harbouring
malicious intent. In the moment of conscious awareness, you
may have noticed the presence of others in the vicinity, or
any exit routes for a potential retreat.

Mastering environmental and situational awareness can
enhance our capacity for assessment, so that we can make
more rapid and confident decisions: whether to engage
or withdraw. Occasionally we may have enough time for
rational deliberation of solutions, while in other cases, we
must act swiftly, or even instantaneously. Our decisions
can happen on two planes: the intellectual one (akin to
Kahneman's System 2 which was introduced in Chapter 3)
or the instrumental one (akin to Kahneman's System 1).
The intellectual choice is born of real-time reflection, using
our cognitive acumen to navigate the threatening scenario.
On the other hand, the instrumental choice will stem from
reflexes, honed through our prior training or experience.
While our analytical eye scans the environment to feed us
with information about incoming threats, the instinctive
fast-track system triggers robust emotional and physical
responses in order to propel us into action. The more
proficiency we gain using both systems, the more adept we
become in evaluating unfolding situations and reacting in
the safest way possible.

The assessment itself can lead toward three core solutions. If we deem an individual as unthreatening, we can
employ psychological tactics such as de-escalation. If we
fear for our safety, it's wiser to withdraw and seek escape
routes. If neither option is available – for example, when

facing aggression or violence – we most likely need to brace ourselves for a physical exchange.

Confident assessment is essential, as it enables us to act decisively and with conviction. Once we've determined the nature of the situation, we can employ certain techniques and strategies in an attempt to minimize threats and protect ourselves from danger.

Take Aways

- In the process of assessment, we may have limited time to determine the nature of the threat we are facing. We usually will need to act quickly, recognizing the level of danger, noticing the presence of others, and identifying potential exit routes.
- During assessment, we engage our intuitive radar (akin to Kahneman's System 1), or have time to deliberate our options (akin to Kahneman's System 2) in an attempt to determine our next steps.
- A comprehensive grasp of environmental cues, incorporating both analytical and intuitive elements, enhances our proficiency in threat assessment.
- Assessment acumen is derived from previous experience and training.
- Three core choices we face during assessment include employing psychological techniques such as de-escalation, withdrawal and physical defence.

Psychological and Linguistic Techniques

Depending on the level of threat and the type of conflict we face, we can employ a variety of psychological and linguistic techniques to keep ourselves safe. Practising a broad range of these methods can be an incredibly valuable tool, not only in self-defence scenarios, but also in everyday-life situations.

De-Escalation

In Chapter 1: Women's Power, we saw how female police officers handled aggressive individuals using emotional intelligence and de-escalation. When dealing with a situation where retreat or withdrawal isn't our first option (or isn't an option at all), we can employ such strategies for conflict resolution and crisis management, with the aim of minimizing or avoiding physical confrontation. During the process, verbal and non-verbal strategies can be used to defuse an intense situation.

De-escalation can be a slow-burner, as it may take time to reduce an aggressor's state of agitation. However, when seen from a self-defence perspective, it can be an extremely potent weapon in potentially dangerous situations, preventing physical violence whenever possible.

In the process of de-escalation, consider the following steps:

- **Listen:** Try to see if you can determine the source of the person's concerns. Actively listen to what they are saying and try to understand their perspective. This will demonstrate that you are considering their feelings, and it can potentially calm down their emotions. Be patient when waiting for the person to respond, as they may be releasing frustration before they start explaining how they're feeling.
- **Be empathetic:** Offer comments to reflect what the person has just said. This will demonstrate that you understand their concerns. Acknowledging other person's feelings will foster a sense of respect. You can use phrases such as: "I can see why you're upset", "I understand why you're feeling this way", or "I can see your point".
- **Remain calm:** Stay non-aggressive with your words and actions, so as not to provoke the person to resort to

physical violence. Use non-threatening body language and do not shout. Our own composure can have a calming effect on the other person.

- **Communicate well:** Use a clear and calm voice. If you are comfortable to do so, maintain eye contact to connect with the person. You can also nod to express understanding. While staying calm and empathetic, remember to also uphold your boundaries. You want to appear neutral – not aggressive, but not weak either.
- **Offer options:** You can use this strategy to allow the person to think outside of their current state of mind. Ask open-ended questions to get them thinking. This may help decrease their emotional triggers, as they can mentally move away from the source of the problem. It can also make the person feel more in control, and can decrease their need to oppose, or resist.
- **Respect the space:** Try to naturally maintain some physical space between you and the person, in order to effectively communicate while remaining at a safe distance. Avoid touching the other person or coming too close to them.

During the de-escalation process, certain negotiation tactics can also be used. According to Chris Voss, a former FBI hostage negotiator and author, asking open ended questions with a soothing tone of voice is one of the best negotiation tactics. Other methods used in negotiations which can also apply in the de-escalation process include:

- **Labelling and mirroring:** When dealing with an aggressive individual, repeat their words (mirroring), and acknowledge their emotions (labelling). This can help to create a connection and minimize the aggressive behaviour.
- **Accusation audit:** Using this strategy, you address any potential concerns of the individual, before they have

the opportunity to bring them up themselves. In this way, you demonstrate understanding which can help to build trust.[41]

When de-escalating, we want to understand the behaviour and emotional processing of the individual we're dealing with. At times, it may be possible for us to detangle the core issue which caused the individual to become disruptive in the first place. We can offer solutions, if any are possible. This will work on a rational level. What will be happening on an emotional level is quite different – the person is likely to be going through an episode where their thinking brain won't be as activate.

One way of thinking about it is to look into the processing of our brains. Even though we know that the brain is interconnected, we can simplify the anatomy and function of it by dividing it into three main regions: the reptilian brain (the one associated with basic survival instincts), the limbic system (associated with emotions and memory), and the neocortex (connected with thinking and reasoning).

With this simplified model of the human brain in mind, according to security expert Gershon Ben Keren,[42] we can envision the de-escalation process as helping to move the agitated person from their reptilian/limbic system over to their reasoning brain. If an agitated individual starts searching for solutions to the situation, instead of just focusing on their emotions, it can take away their justification for violence.

While this tactic works well in certain scenarios, we need to recognize the limitations of this processing. When an angry individual is triggered by a flush of extreme emotions, it may be difficult for them to calm down, and in some cases, as Keren explains, telling the person to "relax" can actually reverse the process of bringing them to stability, as it may be

---

41 Voss, C, *Never Split the Difference: Negotiating as if Your Life Depended on It*, Random House Business Books, 2017
42 www.bostonkravmaga.com/kravmagaboston-media.html

interpreted as posturing (a display of dominance from us). If the reptilian part of their brain perceives our direct message as an order, or a threat, they can respond with aggression. Therefore, it's important to bear in mind our own body language and non-verbal processing, which should remain non-threatening. As Voss mentions, "Body language and tone of voice – not words – are our most powerful tools."

When deciding to engage in the de-escalation process in a potentially threatening scenario, you need to keep a few things in mind. Firstly, consider whether or not you have been trained to do this, or whether you have practised this tactic before. If you haven't engaged in a similar situation in the past, ask yourself whether you possess the communication and assertiveness skills needed to face an irate person. You may need to evaluate your own emotional state first before engaging in this strategy – if you aren't ready to face the individual, you probably shouldn't. You can use your instincts to determine whether or not you are ready to use this technique.

You also need to take your physical abilities into account. While de-escalation is widely used by females, be conscious that you may still need to be ready to protect yourself. Being mindful of the aggressor's size and strength can be a determining factor in whether or not you decide to act. Recognizing the presence of other people around you will also be key, as it can provide an extra level of support. In a similar way, you may need to consider your surroundings and potential exit routes to prepare yourself in case the de-escalation fails.

Being ready to defend yourself at any given moment means establishing a solid stance, keeping your distance and using frames (being ready to have your hands extended forward whenever personal space is being threatened) to prevent any possible strikes and physical attacks. The moment someone invades your personal space by cutting distance and threatening you, you are dealing with an assault. From a legal standpoint, in many countries you can pre-emptively attack in this position, if necessary.

Take Aways

- The process of de-escalation can be your first port of call when dealing with an upset or agitated individual. The aim is to calm the situation down, minimize the threat and avoid the situation resulting in violence if possible.
- The process of de-escalation involves techniques such as listening, empathizing, seeking solutions, and communicating in a non-aggressive way.
- De-escalation is similar to a negotiation process, where you're trying to find a peaceful solution to the problem, using strategies such as mirroring and labelling.
- In the process of de-escalation, our aim is to take the person away from an agitated state (where their limbic system is largely activated) into a state where they have to involve their thinking brain.
- During the process of de-escalation, your priority should always be on protecting yourself. If the de-escalation tactic doesn't offer the desired result, it's best to disengage and seek help or exit routes.

Sociolinguistic Convergence

Sociolinguistic convergence is a cheeky way to make ourselves more likeable. It's the ability to modify our language in order to "align" ourselves to the person we're communicating with. It can involve tactics such as changing our vocabulary, pronunciation, accent, tone of voice, or even aligning our non-verbal communication – mimicking someone's body language – to make ourselves more similar to our interlocutor.

I guarantee that you've seen sociolinguistic convergence at play more than you think you have. Imagine that you know a person who left Scotland a long time ago and has been living in the US for the last ten years. They may have progressively picked up the North American accent during their time living in America, yet when visiting their home town in Scotland, or when they are interacting with friends and family, they seemingly very easily switch back to their original Scottish accent.

The convergence process often happens on a subconscious level, without our rational awareness. It's a process that has broad psychological implications, as it can help us build rapport and connect with people. Its usage may also stem from the desire to identify with certain local social norms, or the simple desire to be more likeable and accepted.

Sociolinguistic convergence can be a tool that is used during situations of conflict – for example, we could adjust our accent and way of communicating to create a sense of connection. In low-level threat scenarios this can be used to de-escalate and potentially diffuse a tense situation.

Converging your vocabulary and your speech may reduce the perceived social distance between you and the threatening individual. You may appear more "familiar", creating a perception of closer social distance. The person may become more receptive to your words, and the tone of your voice. Language similarity can make you appear more approachable and non-threatening, indicating that you come from the same background, which in turn can decrease the likelihood of threatening behaviour escalating.

Aligning your language to match your interlocutor's social background will demonstrate respect and understanding. In de-escalation it will be important to create common ground, decreasing the level of hostility, and promoting a sense of understanding.

It's important to note that social convergence has its limitations, and if not expressed authentically and with respect, it can create more tension than there was initially. This tactic should only be used when you feel confident in your language skills. Unease and hesitation, or a forced/fake convergence may be interpreted as a manipulative tactic.

Assertiveness When Dealing with a Predator

When dealing with a potential sexual predator, or a harasser, we have to act confidently in order to stop the attacker in their tracks. We need to employ strong body language, and a firm and assertive tone of voice. These are the verbal and non-verbal weapons that can save us from unwanted advances by acquaintances and strangers alike.

Assertiveness is a style of communication in which you assert your rights and express your opinion. This doesn't have to involve aggression, but it has to be clear, concise and to the point. Assertiveness is usually described as a form of de-escalation, but in the case of a sexual predator, it will be very different from the tactics described previously, in which we stay compassionate and empathetic toward the agitated person. When using the assertiveness tactic against malicious or coercive behaviour, we need to be able to express our disapproval in a firm and convincing manner.

Some examples of the use of assertive language include:

- Saying "no" instead of "I don't think so", and saying it with conviction, asserting your statements confidently without doubting yourself.
- Keeping your statements short, and avoiding over-explaining your decisions.
- If needed, repeating your statement several times to ensure that the listener has heard you and understood.
- Using non-verbal cues to strengthen the message, including shaking your head and keeping a serious demeanour.
- Avoiding apologizing – do not say "sorry". This will imply that you don't feel secure in your decision or opinion, and this may open the door for further probing.

When employed early, and in a safe setting (such as in the presence of other people, or when we're not isolated in a vulnerable context), assertiveness can be extremely effective in allowing us to confidently face and dissolve attempts of coercion and manipulation.

Be conscious that on some occasions, assertiveness as a method of avoiding a dangerous situation may not be enough. If the aggressor is not respecting your wishes, or if you suspect an imminent threat from an attacker, you should aim to employ other strategies. These strategies may include using a raised tone of voice, screaming, and loudly informing anyone in the surrounding area that you are in danger. Being loud may put the attacker off, as he might worry about other people getting involved. You may need to consider immediate withdrawal, or in worst-case scenarios – be prepared to engage in physical defence.

Take Aways

- Verbal tactics and responses differ greatly when we face a sexual predator or a harasser. Employing a soothing tone of voice, empathy and compassion, as discussed in the de-escalation section, will not be helpful in this situation.
- Assertiveness tactics include setting boundaries, clear and confident communication, expressing our concerns and clearly stating our expectations and limits. The aim is to say no in a firm and convincing way.
- When the level of perceived threat escalates, shouting or screaming, preparing for withdrawal or for physical exchange may be your safest options.

Verbal Responses to Threats

Verbal communication during situations of conflict is of utmost importance, particularly in moments pertaining to our safety. The words we choose and how we express ourselves can mean the difference between becoming a victim, or successfully extricating ourselves from harm.

Our verbal cues serve as a voice aimed both toward ourselves, reaffirming our beliefs, and to others, informing them of our boundaries. The ability to communicate clearly and effectively is paramount, especially when faced with situations that may pressure us into actions that go against our values or wishes.

Consider a scenario where your boss invites you for a drink, but you are uncertain about the purpose or objective of the meeting. In such cases, asking open-ended questions will become crucial to gain clarity. Assertively expressing yourself, saying no, or seeking further information will empower you, allow you to establish a sense of control, and enable you to uphold your boundaries. An appropriate response has the power to safeguard you from unwanted advances, unnecessary stress, and potential risks to your safety.

Examples of Assertive Verbal Responses

When verbally communicating with an aggressor or a harasser, we should consider certain non-physical counter-attacks that can be used as deterrents. These could include assertive vocal responses pertaining to your readiness to defend yourself, threatening the attacker about the consequences of their actions, notifying the aggressor that you have taken action toward safety, or mentioning a person of authority you can turn to for help. You can also warn the harasser of any bystanders and witnesses who are present, or mention that you're ready to identify the aggressor to other parties. Depending on the level of perceived threat, consider some of the following responses:

Low-Level Threat Scenarios

"I will not tolerate this behaviour."

"Stop harassing me. I will report your behaviour if you don't stop."

"Stay back, I know how to defend myself."

"Back off, or you will regret the consequences."

"This stops now, or I will notify the police."

"Stop, or I will call security."

Moderate- to High-Level Threat Scenarios

"Back off! Leave me alone!"

"Stay away from me!"

"I'm warning you to stay back!"

"Call the police!"

"There is a witness watching us, you're not getting away."

"I just called the emergency services and the police are tracking my location."

"I have taken photos of you, and the authorities will have them if anything happens to me."

"I will remember your face, your voice, and everything about you."

"I texted this location to my boyfriend, and he knows I'm with you."

"I know who you are, and you're not going to get away with this if anything happens to me."

(For sexually motivated assaults): "I am HIV positive, think twice."

* * *

Apart from the words that we use, we should also pay attention to the quality of our voice as we speak. Depending on the context, you may need to use a stronger or more assertive tone of voice, especially when standing your ground and establishing your boundaries.

Here are some examples of how you can use paralinguistics (the vocal aspect of your communication) in boundary assertion when someone invades your personal space:

- **Tone of voice:** In low-level threat scenarios, be assertive yet calm. Use a firm voice to convey that you are serious without sounding aggressive or angry. If the situation escalates, the tone of your voice can become more demanding or threatening.
- **Volume:** Depending on the context, you can use a lower voice to inform the person of their invasion of your space, or raise your voice to indicate more seriousness.
- **Pause:** Leave spaces between your phrases so that the listener can process the given information. This allows them time to understand the importance of the message. This use of paralinguistics is applicable for low-level threat scenarios.
- **Intonation:** Emphasize certain words or phrases that indicate boundary setting. For example, highlight the words "appreciate" and "personal space" in a sentence such as: "I would appreciate if you gave me some personal space."
- **Pitch:** Using a low-pitched voice can help indicate seriousness. A deeper voice may give off the impression of confidence and assertiveness.

The examples given show how certain qualities of our voice can be used, in conjunction with other non-verbal cues, to convey a message. It is essential to gauge the seriousness of a given situation and to adjust our communication accordingly. The perception of our confidence will be influenced by a spectrum of cues, such as facial expressions, body language, and the words we choose to use.

Take Aways

- Verbal communication is crucial when assertively expressing ourselves, and protecting our boundaries. It is also key to effectively extracting ourselves from dangerous situations.
- Strong verbal skills equip us with a better sense of control, confidence and self-assurance.
- Exercising a good vocal response that is relevant to the level of threat we may find ourselves faced with can be helpful for in-the-moment support.
- Using paralinguistics, which is the vocal aspect of our communication, including the tone and pitch of our voice, can greatly improve the quality of our messaging.

Self-Talk

Another communication tool which we can use in situations where our safety may be at risk, is strong and positive internal self-talk. This is the internal dialogue we have within ourselves, encompassing our thoughts, beliefs and interpretations. This inner talk shapes the perceptions we have of ourselves, and influences our emotions and mindset. Whether conscious or pre-conditioned, self-talk has the power to impact various aspects of our lives, including decision-making, resilience and self-esteem.

You have probably experienced inner dialogue in various forms, including positive self-talk (motivational and supportive), or negative self-talk (possibly derived from past traumatic experiences or conditioning). There are also other forms of inner dialogue, including instructional self-talk (which provides guidance in specific situations – for example, when we try to command ourselves to relax) and rational self-talk (using reasoning for problem solving and maintaining objectivity – for example, "He didn't really mean it, you are being triggered from past experience.")

Monitoring our automatic self-talk, which operates at a subconscious level, can unveil a lot, including patterns of thoughts and beliefs. In his book *What to Say When You Talk to Your Self*,[43] bestselling author and respected behavioural researcher Shad Helmstetter sheds light on the profound effects of self-talk on our bodies and self-perception. Helmstetter explains how self-talk significantly influences our perception of societal roles, as well as our actions, feelings and behaviours. Personally, I have found self-talk to be an invaluable tool in cultivating a positive relationship with myself, in excelling at work, and when motivating myself for physical exercise. I've also used Helmstetter's audio books extensively with great results – they always give my assertiveness a big boost and infuse me with positive energy for constructive action.

Do you recall situations when you said to yourself, "Let's do it!" or "I've got this!"? This is a perfect example of how positive self-talk can guide us toward taking necessary actions in an empowered and constructive way.

When combined with strong body language and a confident tone of voice, positive self-talk can truly become a powerful asset in managing conflicts and high-stress scenarios, and in enhancing our levels of self-esteem. When faced with a potential threat, mentally reaffirming our strengths and empowering ourselves to take action will be invaluable.

It is important to practise positive self-talk regularly, so that it becomes part of our belief system. Everyday practice can greatly boost our self-esteem and perceived level of confidence.

Examples of Self-Talk During Stranger Approach
Imagine you are taking the last train home, and a stranger is approaching you on an otherwise deserted platform. He is

---

43 Helmstetter, S, *What to Say When You Talk to Your Self*, Gallery Books, 2017

acting unusually, and your instincts inform you that this may be an uncomfortable interaction.

Some of the self-talk you can employ in that moment may include:

- Repeating phrases such as: "Stay calm, I can do this, I can control my emotions", "I've been here before", "I am fully aware and capable".
- Asserting your strengths: "I am strong", "I can run if needed", "I know how to position myself for safety".
- Reminding yourself: "Safety is my priority", "If he continues to engage, I will communicate my boundaries VERY clearly", "I will fight back if needed".
- Saying things like: "There is help if I need it", "I can use my voice to call for help".

* * *

You can practise self-talk each time you find yourself in a conflict situation with friends, family or at work. Make sure that your inner dialogue is strong and confident. Pay close attention to the words that you use, to make sure they don't undermine your abilities or skills. Self-talk is all about believing in yourself and your capabilities, while remaining objective and realistic.

Strategies for Safe Withdrawal

Imagine you're in a potentially threatening situation, and your assessment is guiding you toward withdrawal. It could be a moment when your inner voice urges you to make a quick exit, to step away from a tense conversation, or run to safety. Depending on the circumstances and the environment, these retreat options may vary in terms of ease and effectiveness.

There are times when asserting your boundaries and simply removing yourself from a situation might suffice. But, in the presence of a physical threat, retreat needs to happen with awareness and caution. This is where our environmental assessment becomes absolutely crucial. Think of this assessment as your personal radar, always feeding you with vital information about your surroundings – your distance from the potential threat, and the safest paths you can take for a swift escape.

When escaping, it's crucial to identify the most-accessible exit routes and the nearest zones of safety. These are usually the places where you will find other people, like shops or residential buildings. Your best bet is to avoid confined spaces where you could get trapped, and instead to aim for areas with plenty of open space, so you're not backed into a corner. Take note of any potential dead-end streets where you might find yourself boxed in. Having a good grasp of the local geography can make a big difference to your escape plan. If you do, however, end up in a tight spot, use doors, windows and emergency exits wherever possible to help make your exit smoother.

Additionally, when trying to steer clear of physical confrontation, you can use certain personal safety tools. Consider carrying a personal safety alarm which can trigger a 140 dB noise when released. Throwing objects can also create a distraction to buy you some time. If there are obstacles like furniture or other large barriers, use them to slow down the attacker.

Your voice can also be used as a weapon – screaming and shouting can catch your attacker off guard and draw attention to the situation, possibly prompting people nearby to step in.

In situations where your shouting is to no avail, or when you find yourself isolated with the attacker, you can temporarily pretend to comply, in order to de-escalate the situation. This gives you a chance to assess your surroundings, spot escape routes, or wait for a better opportunity to resist or make your getaway.

Self-Distancing

In the context of self-defence, self-distancing refers to the act of creating physical and emotional space between ourselves and potentially dangerous individuals or groups. It involves implementing strategies to minimize harm and prioritize our safety. This proactive measure includes adjusting our positioning, utilizing barriers, and firmly maintaining personal boundaries. By creating distance, we gain a greater sense of control over the situation, and are better able to establish potential escape routes.

Examples of Self-Distancing on Public Transport
Lauren often commutes on public buses. One day, she notices a man on her bus who looks suspicious and makes her feel uncomfortable. In order to ensure her own safety without getting emotionally involved in the situation, Lauren takes precautionary measures. She decides to employ some self-distancing techniques:

- She changes where she is sitting on the bus, to reduce the risk of potential harm.
- She uses physical barriers to position herself for safety. She may choose to sit nearer to other passengers, or closer to the exit.
- When her personal space is being threatened, Lauren assertively communicates her need for physical distance.
- Lauren refrains from engaging with the individual by remaining calm and composed, avoiding direct eye contact and using her peripheral vision to screen her surroundings. By disengaging with the individual, Lauren can minimize her chances of having to interact with the stranger.

Please note that these distancing techniques have to go hand-in-hand with constant monitoring of the surroundings, trusting your instincts and seeking assistance and help from others around you when necessary.

Examples of Self-Distancing During a Social Gathering

Helen is at a work event in a crowded space. She notices an individual who is behaving unusually. In order to create distance between herself and the individual, she takes precautionary measures:

- She positions herself away from the individual, seeking open spaces. If necessary, Helen will relocate to another part of the room.
- She engages with other people, such as friends or work colleagues, and joins them in a conversation, in order to discourage any advances from the stranger, thus decreasing the likelihood of the individual approaching her.
- Helen remains calm, keeps an upright posture, and avoids prolonged eye contact.
- If the individual decides to approach her, Helen will use assertive statements such as, "I am not interested, please keep your distance."
- If the individual continues to disregard her wishes and disrespect her boundaries, Helen will seek assistance from others nearby.

Take Aways

- Practising situational awareness is the best way to identify exit routes and places we can run toward for safety.
- Avoid dead-ends, and confined spaces, as this limits your retreat options. Wherever possible, aim for large, empty spaces.
- You can use a personal safety alarm or your voice to distract the attacker and attract attention.
- Using barriers or throwing objects to give you time to run to safety can be beneficial during a retreat.

- When everything else fails and you are faced with an attacker, faking compliance may give you enough time to explore alternative exit routes and ways to run to safety.
- Self-distancing can be a great way to remove yourself quietly from a situation.

Fight or Flight – Bodily Reactions to Stress

When we're in the middle of a heated argument or feel like danger is looming, our bodies kick into action, entering what is commonly referred to as "fight or flight" mode. Researchers describe these states as hyperarousal or an acute stress response. In these moments, a few things can happen. Our bodies can prepare for a physical defence – the state of "fight". We may also experience an urge to run toward safety in order to escape or avoid the impending threat – this is the "flight" reaction. However, in the middle of all this, something different can sometimes happen – we might suddenly find ourselves gripped by fear and anxiety, feeling immobilized and temporarily stuck. This state of momentarily paralysis is referred to as the "freeze" state.

How we react to danger is influenced by various factors, including our personal past experiences, our individual personalities, and the severity of the threat itself. The states we enter during confrontation can also be transient, as an individual initially in the freeze state can transition into the flight mode.

The heightened stress response, which can also be observed in the animal kingdom, has always been there to protect us from immediate danger from predators. In the modern world, however, this response may also get activated in non-physically threatening scenarios – for example, when we experience stress at work, or before an important meeting or event. Learning how to deal with such heightened states can equip us with the capacity to calm ourselves down when a threat isn't actually present, but also when we prepare ourselves to deal with a genuine threat to our safety.

* * *

Many things happen in our bodies in the moment when we perceive a threat. The brain sends signals to the body, preparing it for action. The sympathetic nervous system gets activated, leading to the release of stress hormones – including adrenaline and noradrenaline – into the bloodstream. This results in an increased heart rate, which pumps more blood and oxygen into the muscles and organs. Our pupils dilate to enhance our vision, our lungs open up to allow for more oxygen intake, our blood pressure rises and our sensory perception is heightened. If you've ever noticed your body entering this kind of state, with your heart racing during a moment of high-level stress, you've likely experienced the fight-or-flight response.

Having our bodies primed for action when faced with a perceived threat can be a blessing, but when we're driven by extreme emotions, we may find ourselves incapable of doing anything at all. Even if we're lucky and we don't actually freeze, hyperarousal can still greatly affect our performance. If you have not trained your mind and body to deal with high levels of stress, your psychological functioning and physiological systems may be impacted to the point that it will feel debilitating. You may not be able to think clearly, and your body won't function effectively.[44] When your heart rate exceeds 115 beats per minute (bpm), you're likely to lose your fine motor skills, and when it ranges between 115 and 160 bpm, your blood flow will be

44 Sorrentino, D, "Impact of the Tach-Psych Effect while under Stress, Duress or Heightened Anxiety!", *International Critical Incident Stress Foundation, Inc.*, icisf.org/impact-of-the-tach-psych-effect-while-under-stress-duress-or-heightened-anxiety/

affected – as blood will mainly be directed toward the major organs, and away from the extremities.

In order to prepare your physical defence when in this state, you need to get your gross motor skills involved, which means you will have less dexterity and coordination, especially in the fingers and hands. Your hands may also be trembling and shaky. If your muscles tense too much, it can interfere with your coordination, preventing you from executing precise movements. You may also lose your peripheral vision and the capacity to hear what is happening around you. This is referred to as auditory occlusion. What's more, you're likely to lose the ability to process information. This usually happens when your heart rate is above 160 bpm; at this point, you will struggle to think clearly and may have difficulties in problem solving.

Unless you can control your heart rate, the hyperarousal state can take over and paralyse you, meaning that you will potentially be unable to deal with the situation. It's paramount, therefore, that we actively seek ways in which we can better react to stressful situations. By using a variety of techniques, including breathing and the practice of mindfulness, we can start to change our reactions, and stay in charge of our cognitive and physical processing during situations of conflict.

Take Aways

- During high-level conflict situations, our bodies can react by entering the state of "fight or flight", also referred to as hyperarousal or acute stress response.
- During hyperarousal our bodies prepare for conflict by producing performance-boosting hormones that equip us with more blood and oxygen, facilitating a retreat (flight state), or bracing us for a physical exchange (fight state). When the stress response is accompanied by extreme emotions, such as fear and anxiety, we can also

experience the state of "freeze", which makes us feel paralysed and unable to move.

- Heightened states of stress can lead to impaired motor skills, which can have an impact on how well we're able to defend ourselves. High stress can also cause the inability to process information.
- Learning how to calm our nervous system down when our heart rate is high can be crucial in regulating our emotions, and protecting us from entering the freeze state.

Calming Down with Breathing

Every day, we naturally take 12–16 breaths per minute, most of the time without even thinking about it. It's usually only during periods of high stress or intense physical exertion that we become aware of our respiration. In those moments, our breath becomes sharper, and impossible to ignore. At times, our sympathetic nervous system will trigger the fight-or-flight response, preparing us for action. As mentioned previously, this reaction can be paralysing and strip us of the mental and physical control over our bodies. To counteract this, and to restore balance, we need to be able to activate our parasympathetic nervous system in order to calm down. Without this knowledge, we are likely to sweat, panic and lose control.

Breath education will be applicable not just in threatening scenarios, but also in our everyday lives, including in social interactions and at work. The ability to regulate our breath will empower us to effectively cope with stress, enhance our overall quality of life, and promote awareness and focus.

The following exercise will guide you through activating the parasympathetic nervous system, in which your heart rate is likely to slow down. You can employ this breathing method when faced with a challenging situation, and within a very short period of time you are likely to recognize the benefits of this practice. Once you get accustomed to this form of breathing, it will be a strong component of your confidence toolbox when dealing with conflicts and highly stressful scenarios. Having this heart-rate-relief technique up your sleeve will also bring you a greater sense of control and trust in your ability for emotional regulation.

The principle of this breathing method is to extend the exhalations, making them longer than the inhalations.

EXERCISE: PARASYMPATHETIC BREATHING

- Take a deep breath in through the nose on the count of three (2–4 seconds) then exhale on the count of six (4–6 seconds). You can exhale either through the nose, or through the mouth. When breathing out through the mouth, it may be helpful to create a slight constriction at the back of your throat, to slow down the exhale.
- You can further extend the breath counts, for example, to four counts on the inhale and eight counts on the exhale.
- Continue breathing in this manner for few minutes and notice your body becoming calmer.

Take Away

- Acquiring the skill of breathing to activate the para-sympathetic nervous system can assist us in effectively navigating stressful situations, and can foster a greater sense of control, equilibrium, and both mental and physical stability.

Conclusion

While facing conflict isn't easy, as there may be various threats present during a confrontation, there are effective ways in which we can respond when dealing with difficult and stressful scenarios. Being aware of our surroundings and being able to process information will be key, as this will allow us to assess and mitigate risks early on. An accurate assessment of the situation, both on an intellectual and an instinctive level, can prove crucial when deciding on the best course of action to be taken in a given moment.

Our intuitive radars, past experiences and training can guide us toward different solutions, such as employing psychological and linguistic tools, assertiveness tactics, or safely withdrawing from a situation. When aiming to calm a situation down or help an upset person to regain stability, we can use de-escalation tactics. On the other hand, when dealing with a sexual predator or harasser, assertiveness tactics will be the best tools to use to save ourselves.

While employing these methods and strategies, it's important to recognize their potential risks and limitations, and, above all, to always prioritize our safety.

As we step into the conflict arena, our bodies can slip into a state of hyperarousal, bracing for a physical fight or a retreat. These states can be debilitating, and can affect our physical performance and diminish our cognitive functioning. It is therefore important to remember that we have the ability to calm our nervous systems down, and that this can help us immensely when dealing with stress.

CHAPTER 5
PHYSICAL DEFENCE

"Attack where his spirit is lax, throw him into confusion, irritate and terrify him. Take advantage of the enemy's rhythm when he is unsettled and you can win."
—Miyamoto Musashi

When it comes to physical defence, there are a few important things to keep in mind, both for your safety and from a legal standpoint. There are many guidebooks out there that show pretty dazzling self-defence tactics, but some of them are unrealistic, and a few might even get you Into trouble with the law.

Watching action films can make it all seem a bit confusing too, as these blur the lines between what's actually practical in real life, and what's just movie magic. As we've seen in earlier chapters, certain situations can impair our motor skills and judgement, so it is therefore essential to keep a level head and to use common-sense measures when things get physical.

Firstly, you should find out what is considered legally acceptable self-defence in your jurisdiction. You want to make sure that whatever you do falls within the bounds of what's proportionate and necessary. Whether you're defending yourself, others, or your property, what's considered as reasonable can vary from place to place. If there happen to be any weapons around, it's crucial to know which ones are legal and when you can use them. Otherwise, you might find yourself facing assault charges.

Once you're aware of your rights and what's legally acceptable in your jurisdiction, it's time to prepare a practical action plan. This means being mindful of your personal space and learning how to control the distance around you, in order to ward off potential attacks. If distance control doesn't work, and you face a physical threat, this chapter will explain how you can use your body to break free and get away.

You will also be presented with ten different self-defence scenarios that will illustrate a few strategies for dealing with the most common threats.

Law with Regards to Self-Defence

The laws regarding self-defence vary from country to country, but there are certain principles that are common among the western nations.

The general consensus is that you can use reasonable force to protect yourself from imminent physical harm. The force used should be proportional to the perceived threat you are facing. This typically means that the use of force must be justifiable based on the circumstances, and on what you honestly believe is necessary and proportionate given the situation. In some cases, even if your belief turns out to be wrong, you can still be excused in a court of law, as long as you did only what you felt was truly necessary in order to address the perceived threat.

While in some places like New York, the law states you should attempt to retreat and escape the threat wherever possible before resorting to physical violence, in many other places this is still advisable, but it is not a legal requirement. For example, in countries such as the UK, Canada, France, Germany and Poland there is no legal obligation to retreat, and each case is assessed on an individual basis to determine whether or not the force used was reasonable given the circumstances.

The law allowing the use of force (including deadly force) in public when faced with imminent danger, without there being an obligation to escape or retreat, is often referred to as "stand your ground". Even though "stand your ground" is oftentimes portrayed in a way that indicates that the escalation to deadly force is justified in every case, the principle of proportionality still applies. There still needs to be a reasonable belief that there was a necessity to use such force in order to prevent imminent death or great bodily harm.

In some cases, using a pre-emptive strike in self-defence can also apply. When faced with an imminent threat to life or grievous body harm, you don't have to wait for the assailant to attack you first, you can pre-emptively act, using proportionate force.

* * *

When it comes to defending your home or property, in many jurisdictions there are laws allowing the use of force when protecting your place of residence. In the UK, Canada and Australia, reasonable force is allowed in these circumstances. In South Africa, you can also defend your home and property, including the use of deadly force. In the US, there is a "castle doctrine", also commonly referred to as the "make my day" law, which allows individuals to use force (including deadly force) when dealing with a home invasion. In this case, lethal force can be applied to trespassers in order to prevent death or harm to the homeowner, without the need to retreat.[45] If you remember

---

45 "Self-Defense and 'Stand Your Ground'", *National Conference of State Legislatures*, 2023, www.ncsl.org/civil-and-criminal-justice/self-defense-and-stand-your-ground

the movie *Sudden Impact* with the character "Dirty Harry" (played by Clint Eastwood) saying, "Go ahead, make my day", you may recall that this phrase was used in reference to the state of Colorado passing a law that protected people from criminal liability when using force against an intruder in their home.

Apart from protecting ourselves and our properties, in many western countries it's also permittable to use force when defending others if there's a reasonable belief that they are facing an imminent threat or physical harm.

On most occasions, when you adhere to the principle of acting reasonably in the circumstances, without retaliating or attempting to teach someone a lesson, you should be safe from facing criminal charges.

Given the variations in legal principles between countries and regions, though, it's a good idea to familiarize yourself with the fundamental principles governing your jurisdiction. This knowledge can provide you with confidence in your actions when using self-defence, both for your own protection and that of others. You can find this information on your government website, local online legal databases, and local law-enforcement websites. When in doubt, you can visit legal aid organizations, or consult a local attorney.

Weapons Used in Self-Defence

In many places, when you are in immediate danger, you have the right to defend yourself, without weapons, using reasonable force. However, the rules about using weapons can differ widely from one place to another. Some countries and regions might allow things like pepper spray, Tasers or stun guns for self-defence, but there could still be age limits, or only very specific situations in which you're allowed to use these kinds of weapons. When it comes to deadly weapons such as firearms, you are usually required to have a special permit or licence to use these, and you can typically only use them if you're facing a serious and immediate threat, like the risk of death or serious harm.

In the United States, for example, you can generally use firearms for self-defence, but this is subject to state and federal laws. In the UK, most weapons, including pepper spray, are illegal. However, you can use makeshift weapons as long as you're not carrying them with the intent to cause harm. These improvised tools can come in handy when you're facing an immediate threat. For example, using an umbrella or your house keys to fend off a street attacker are both viable options.

If you're looking to equip yourself with self-defence tools, consider purchasing a personal safety alarm, or a spray that is legally accepted in your jurisdiction. For example, the DNA criminal identifier spray is one of the latest innovations that can help catch muggers and thieves. Each spray bottle contains a solution with a unique code which can be linked directly to you or the item you are trying to protect from theft, such as a bicycle or a vehicle.

When sprayed on the perpetrator, the DNA solution will mark them with a UV-detected substance, which can remain on the skin for a few weeks, and up to a few months on clothing. This way, when a suspect is apprehended by the police, it becomes very easy to check whether they have been sprayed by your solution. There are other, more affordable versions of this type of deterrent, including a red gel criminal identifier spray, which will leave marks on the attacker and their clothing for about a week, but which won't be linked to you through a unique DNA code.

* * *

The use (or not) of weapons will largely depend on the context of the situation. If you're protecting your property, you should consider using all legal weapons available. When defending yourself in the street, think about weapons of opportunity that you may have on you: any type of spray, a personal safety alarm, anything that you're carrying with you such as keys, or objects that can be used for striking. When you find yourself in a confined space, you can use any objects available in the surrounding area to create barriers and shields. Always remember that using weapons has to be objectively reasonable given the circumstances. If you fear for your life or that serious harm may be done, use what you believe is necessary to protect yourself.

Controlling Your Personal Space

One of the most crucial elements of de-escalation and self-defence in general is controlling distance. Stepping back and staying at least at arm's length from a potentially threatening individual is key, and at times you may need to frame your arms in front of you to guard your personal space. When facing an attacker one-on-one, it's imperative that we position ourselves for safety by using a defensive stance. This not only signals our unwillingness to engage in combat, but also prepares us to defend against physical advances and potential strikes.

A solid defensive stance involves proper foot positioning, with one leg in front and the other toward the back. Most people have a personal preference for their stance, choosing which foot to place forward for better balance. If you are right-hand dominant, adopting a stance with your left foot in front can be advantageous for preparing to use your rear hand and leg for strikes.

When adopting a defensive stance with your legs apart, extend your hands forward and position your forearms to face the attacker. This arm positioning is generally referred to as a "frame" and it helps control distance, preventing the attacker from invading your personal space. It also enables you to block and shield the upper body from strikes, including punches, slaps and hair-pulls. Your arm frame serves as your standing guard, also allowing you to deflect strikes, push the attacker away, and strike when necessary.

In some situations, you may also need to use your legs to defend yourself from the attacker. For example, when you find yourself on the ground, with your back to the floor and the attacker standing or closing distance from the top position, you can elevate your legs, creating a so called "leg guard" which acts as a defensive shield. The leg guard has various applications, including controlling distance and acting as a frame to protect from strikes. It can be used as an offensive tool to clinch, off-balance the attacker, and also to sweep and strike. Using the leg guard can be very effective, especially when a smaller person is defending against a bigger opponent, as it leverages a stronger part of the body for both defence and offence.

When protecting your personal space, don't forget to use your voice to clearly communicate to the attacker that you won't tolerate their behaviour. You can threaten to defend yourself, including with the use of weapons, or inform the attacker about the consequences of their actions.

Body as a Weapon

When you find yourself in a situation where the attacker is not respecting your personal space and is disregarding your vocal responses, such as warnings to move back, you will likely need to use your body to defend yourself. These types of scenarios can occur in various public situations, such as in the street or at a social gathering. Always rely on common sense and intuition to assess the intentions of the person approaching you and when to take action. When the threat is imminent and you have no exit routes, it's time to push the attacker away or strike.

When in a standing position, it's advisable to initiate attacks using the limb positioned at the rear – either the rear leg or the rear hand. This allows for greater momentum, enhanced torque, and results in more powerful strikes.

For self-defence purposes, particularly when facing a larger and stronger opponent, some of the safest and most effective striking options include:

Knees and elbows: These are among the strongest structures in our anatomy and they can deliver powerful strikes. Knee strikes to the groin area are one of the most potent techniques you can use when defending yourself against a male attacker. When using elbows, you have various options: vertical strikes (eg, raising the elbow to strike beneath the chin), horizontal strikes (hitting the side of the jaw), and rotating elbows (effective when striking from the side or from behind the opponent). Depending on your positioning, these elbow strikes can target the jaw, groin or the attacker's abdomen, which are the most vulnerable areas to attack with the elbow.

Palm strike: Positioning the heel of your palm beneath the attacker's chin or nose can unbalance them, shifting their body weight toward the back and twisting their spine. This can create an opportunity for follow-up attacks, such as knee or foot strikes to the groin. This method is often safer than using a closed fist, as it avoids putting stress on your knuckles, reducing the risk of fracturing your own bones.

Heel strikes: Heel strikes can be highly effective when targeting the knee joint from various angles, including while standing (usually from a side position) and from the ground (when you're lying on your back). When attacking from the ground (while the opponent is standing), or when you're facing away from the attacker (eg, if the attacker has you in a rear bear hug), you can also use heel strikes to target the groin area.

Fist: One of the most effective uses of a closed fist is striking the groin area. When you find yourself in situations where traditional strikes are not an option (eg, when an attacker has locked your hands in a bear hold from behind), using the fist at an angle can be an effective way to target vulnerable areas.

Fingers: In situations where you are pinned against a wall or on the floor, making it difficult to use common striking techniques, fingers can be invaluable. They can be used for throat attacks, eye gouging, pressing thumbs into the attacker's eye sockets, or for twisting the ears. These techniques are considered last-resort solutions and can be highly effective when dealing with an attacker who has confined you to a challenging position from which it is difficult to escape.

Ten Self-Defence Techniques

To picture scenarios in which you may need to employ physical defence, such as escaping from chokes and pins, consider the following examples. The illustrations demonstrate the use of a defensive stance, using appropriate body parts for striking and targeting specific areas of the attacker's body.

When practising these defensive moves with a partner, progressively increase your speed and intensity as you carry them out. For an added challenge, consider starting with your eyes closed, and opening them during the moment of physical contact (when your partner is attacking). By adding the element of surprise, you can better practise your reflex reactions.

Techniques from Standing

Technique 1: Two-on-One Wrist Grab Escape (Overhand Grip)

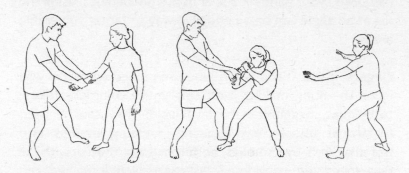

Intro: Someone pulls your arm, locking both of their hands on top of your wrist and forearm.

Step 1: Take a step back with the leg that is opposite to the hand being pulled (eg, if your right hand is being pulled, step back with your left leg), creating a side angle to the attacker holding you. Make sure both of your feet are steady on the ground, with heels planted on the floor, resembling a surf stance.

Step 2: Bring your free hand to the hand being pulled through the gap between the attacker's forearms, from the top. Bring both of your palms together perpendicularly, folding the tops of the fingers to create a strong grip. For a stronger break, bring your front elbow closer toward your front hip while taking a small step forward.

Step 3: Pull the bottom elbow up vertically to break the grip.

Step 4: As soon as the grip breaks, create space by moving away from the attacker, framing your hands in front of your face.

Depending on the context in which the wrist grab occurs, it can also be broken using foot and knee strikes to the groin, or by using a heel to strike the attacker's knee. Strikes can also be used in conjunction with the technical break described.

Technique 2: Double Wrist Grab Escape (Underhand Grip)

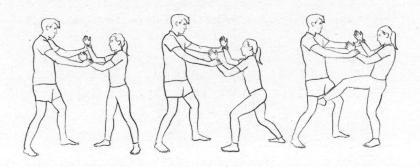

Intro: Someone holds both of your wrists with an underhand grip.

Step 1: Step your dominant leg back to widen your stance, and prepare for a foot/knee strike. Always position your striking leg behind you.

Step 2: Strike the groin with your foot, bringing your rear leg toward the front. Or, strike the groin with your knee, bringing your rear leg toward the front. If there is more distance between you and the attacker, it may be easier to hit with the foot. From closer range, it will be easier to hit with the knee.

While there are other forms of break for this type of wrist grab which do not involve strikes, they may be difficult to perform on a bigger person, and therefore may put you in a potentially vulnerable and unstable position. In a threatening context, where hitting is a reasonable use of force, it is usually safer and more effective to opt for groin strikes.

Technique 3: Standing Front Choke Escape

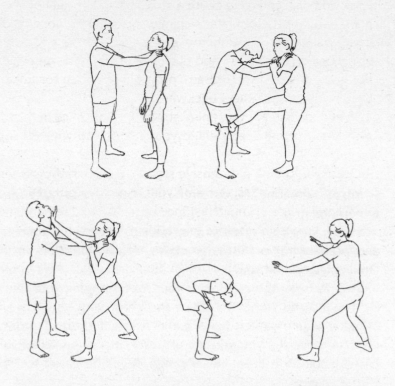

Intro: From a front standing position, someone puts their hands on your throat, creating compression at the neck.

Step 1: Step your dominant leg back and widen your feet, if needed, to establish a solid foundation. Simultaneously, bring both of your hands on top of the attacker's wrists while pulling your elbows downward. This action will help alleviate some of the tension on the neck. Use the attacker's hands as posts for added balance, as if you were hanging onto two branches of a tree.

Step 2: Depending on the distance between you and the attacker, either use your rear leg to deliver a knee strike to the groin, or use your rear leg to deliver a foot strike to the groin.

Step 3: Disengage your dominant hand from the attacker's wrist and proceed to execute a strike using the heel of your palm beneath the attacker's chin, or below their nose. Your hand will travel through the gap between the attacker's arms. Use an open palm and push diagonally to disrupt their posture. Aim for a straight-arm position, to create torque on their spine, forcing them backward.

When executing the palm strike with your right hand, position your right leg behind you to enhance your driving force.

Step 4: Establish a defensive stance, and push the person away with your hands, or frame your hands in front of you.

Step 5: Create as much distance between yourself and the attacker as possible before executing a retreat.

NOTE: You may find it necessary to repeat certain steps or utilize a combination of techniques to successfully break free.

Step 2 and Step 3 can be performed in any sequence. If the choke isn't fully on, you can start with the palm strike. Alternatively, if you are concerned about disconnecting your hand from the attacker's wrist, you can choose to use a series of successive knee strikes to the groin.

Technique 4: Front Bear Hug Escape

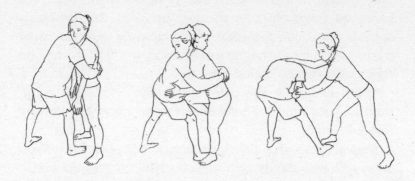

Intro: Someone holds you around the waist from the front, pinning both of your arms.

Step 1: Position the heels of your palms in front of the attacker's hips with your fingers pointing outward, creating a strong frame by connecting your elbows to your pelvis. Simultaneously, step your dominant leg back, pushing your hips away and toward the rear.

Step 2: Execute a strike to the groin, bringing the rear knee forward.

Step 3: Position yourself in a defensive stance before the retreat, framing your hands in front of you and pushing the attacker away if needed.

NOTE: You may find it necessary to repeat Step 2 multiple times to successfully break away. You may also need to switch your leg positioning and strike with your other leg, if the knee strike on your dominant side proves ineffective due to the angle at which the person is standing.

Technique 5: Back Bear Hug Escape

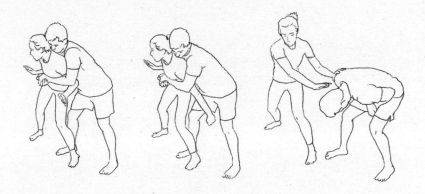

Intro: Someone holds you around the waist from the back, pinning both of your arms.

Step 1: Shift your hips to the side while maintaining a stable stance with your feet apart, to ensure good balance.

Step 2: Form a fist with one hand and strike the groin area, fully extending your arm behind you.

Step 3: Move away safely by pushing the person away, or by framing your hands, before executing a retreat.

NOTE: To break away effectively, you may need to use multiple strikes. Along with the fist strike, think about adding elbow strikes directed at the abdomen or belly region.

Technique 6: Escaping a Double Hand Pin Against the Wall

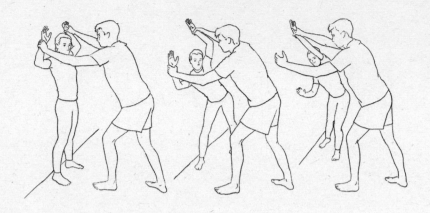

Intro: Someone pins both of your wrists to the wall, facing you.

Step 1: Strike with your knee into the groin.

Step 2: Move your hips to the side to off-pressure the wrist pin.

Step 3: If needed, repeat step number one before retreating.

Technique 7: Escaping from a Single Hand Choke Against the Wall

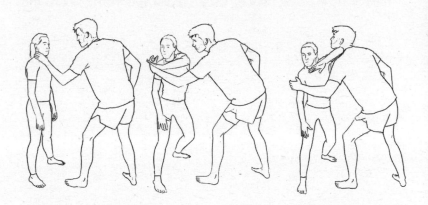

Intro: Someone pins you against the wall with one hand around your throat.

Step 1: Establish a solid base by widening your stance, or bending the knees slightly if necessary. Position the heel of your palm to face the wrist that is choking you.

Step 2: Use the heel of the palm to deliver a powerful strike to the attacker's wrist. Utilize the rotation of your torso and hips to generate power in this movement. Engage your entire body to turn and break the grip.

Step 3: As the attacker's choking hand moves closer to the wall, use your raised elbow to deliver a strike in the opposite direction, aiming for a powerful horizontal hit to the attacker's chin area.

NOTE: Using strikes to the groin is also a feasible option, provided the space between you and the attacker allows for it. Usually, being pressed against the wall means that executing a groin strike effectively may be difficult, due to the restricted potential for forward movement, especially if the attacker is closing the distance. You may also consider using a palm strike to the face (similar to the standing front choke escape). Yet, in a close-range scenario with your feet parallel, this technique may prove to be less effective.

Ground Techniques

Technique 8: Using the Leg Guard to Escape from the Ground

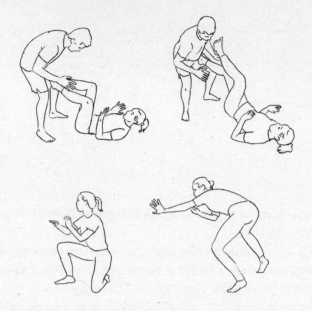

Intro: You find yourself on the ground, with a person approaching you from standing.

Step 1: Use your legs as your guard: raise your feet, externally rotate your knees and toes. Keep your feet positioned toward the attacker's hips as a frame.

Step 2: Execute strikes to the knee area using your heel.

Step 3: Deliver strikes to the groin using your heel.

Step 4: Position one foot on the attacker's hip, using your foot on their body as leverage. Elevate your hips, using your free leg to strike the attacker's face with your heel.

Step 5: When standing up to retreat, make sure to bring up one knee at a time. Maintain a safe knee positioning, elevating the front knee first, while the other shin remains on the floor.

Step 6: Assume a surf stance while maintaining a hand frame before initiating a retreat.

Technique 9: Tripod Sweep Escape

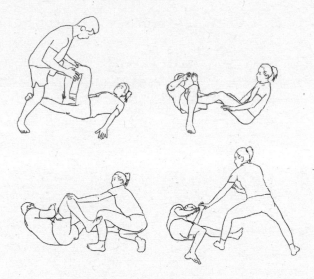

Intro: You are in a lying position with an attacker standing in front of you. The attacker is cutting the distance between you, making your strikes ineffective.

Step 1: Plant one of your feet onto one of the attacker's hips. Hook your hand behind the attacker's ankle, on the same side of their body as your foot is planted. With your second foot, create a "sticky" hook behind their knee on the other leg.

Step 2: Use the three points of leverage to bring the person to the floor: push your foot into their hip, while simultaneously pulling their knee forward with your "sticky" hook and blocking their ankle with your hand.

Step 3: Elevate your torso, bringing your rear shin flat onto the ground. At the same time, lift your front knee and place your front foot firmly on the ground. Put your rear hand onto the ground for a strong base, as you frame with the other hand.

Step 4: Raise your hips, preparing to come into a surf stance.

Step 5: Firmly plant both feet on the ground, maintaining your frame while exiting.

Technique 10: Bridge and Roll Escape from the Mount

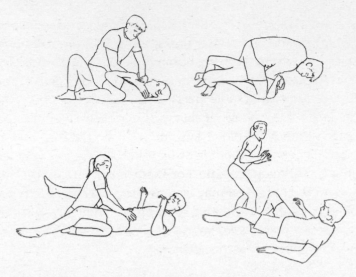

Intro: Someone places both of their hands on your throat while in the mounted position from above you, exerting pressure on your neck.

Step 1: Position your hands on top of the attacker's wrists, pulling your elbows downward. At the same time, bend your knees and draw your heels close toward your hips, with one foot on the floor behind the attacker's ankle to block their movement.

Step 2: Initiate a bridge by pushing your hips diagonally, toward the side of the ankle you have blocked. Perform the bridge at approximately a 45-degree angle (up and to the side), maintaining elevated hips as you roll the person to the side.

Step 3: Upon landing, widen your knees on the floor for a stable base. Lift your torso and frame your hands against their hips, exerting a downward push.

Step 4: Use your hand frame as an anchor point to propel yourself into standing, either by raising one knee at a time, or by jumping into a surf stance in one go.

Step 5: Create distance by moving away while maintaining hand frames for safety.

Conclusion

The scenarios presented in this chapter serve as examples of what you may encounter during a physical confrontation. While they aim to illustrate some basic principles, including remaining steady on your feet, using your body as a weapon and targeting vulnerable parts of an attacker's body, the techniques shown may not always be immediately applicable, as each situation in unique, and you will likely need to employ various different methods in order to effectively free yourself from a threatening scenario. For example, as well as breaking away from a hold, you may also need to execute additional techniques before retreating to safety. Additionally, you may need to use your voice, improvised weapons or barriers to remove yourself from the scenario.

Most importantly, when faced with imminent danger, your fighting spirit will play a major role in getting yourself to safety. Remaining confident in your actions and doing what is necessary with total determination, certainty and commitment will be key in allowing you to escape the threat.

CHAPTER 6
HEALING FROM TRAUMA

"Healing is a matter of time, but it is sometimes also a matter of opportunity."

—Hippocrates

Understanding Trauma and its Impact

Defining Trauma and PTSD

The word "trauma" originates from the Greek term for "wound", and refers to a deeply disturbing event or experience – or a series of events and experiences – which affect(s) a person's ability to cope and function effectively. Trauma can be caused by a range of situations, including physical and emotional abuse, other violence, or the witnessing of a terrible event. Trauma often has a long-lasting effect on an individual's physical and emotional wellbeing.

According to research, trauma can contribute to the development of mental health conditions such as depression, anxiety, and post-traumatic stress disorder (PTSD). Certain forms of trauma, such as sexual violence and domestic abuse, tend to disproportionately affect women more than men. Studies reveal that 78 per cent of women who have experienced physical and sexual violence have also experienced life-threatening trauma, with over a third of these women attempting suicide, and 22 per cent of them engaging in self-harm.[46] Complex trauma can further damage self-esteem and disrupt our sense of self, influencing how we relate to others and how we perceive ourselves. It can also serve as a catalyst for future traumatization and victimization.

Many individuals impacted by trauma develop post-traumatic stress disorder, which manifests in haunting flashbacks and severe anxiety. This condition profoundly affects mental strength, physical vitality and spiritual equilibrium. For those suffering from PTSD, revisiting past experiences can feel life-threatening and harmful. Among women, intimate partner violence, bullying, rape and sexual assault are commonly associated with PTSD. Sexual violence in particular has been identified as a pernicious contributor for developing PTSD, particularly among females.[47]

PTSD often leaves individuals feeling trapped in a state of relentless hypervigilance and perpetual unease, increasing their ability to detect potential threats, as they remain on high alert, constantly anticipating danger. In such a state, distinguishing between a genuine threat and a false alarm becomes increasingly challenging, as the line between reality and illusion becomes blurry.

As we explored in Chapter 1: Women's Power, it is crucial for traumatized individuals to focus on the present and to identify patterns of behaviour and their bodily reactions to stress to help them gain a better understanding of when a threat is real and when it is not.

---

46 Scott, S, MacManus, S, "Hidden Hurt: Violence, Abuse and Disadvantage in the Lives of Women", *DMSS Research for Agenda*, 2016, www. agendaalliance.org/documents/124/Hidden-Hurt-Full-Report.pdf
47 Scott, S, MacManus, S, "Hidden Hurt: Violence, Abuse and Disadvantage in the Lives of Women", *DMSS Research for Agenda*, 2016, www. agendaalliance.org/documents/124/Hidden-Hurt-Full-Report.pdf

Given the arduous task of healing from trauma-related conditions, various approaches may prove helpful. The tools described in the following sections not only offer guidance on how to help resolve trauma, but also hold significant importance in terms of personal safety, aiding in the prevention of potential future victimization.

The Psychological Wound: Exploring the Internal Impact

Dr Gabor Maté, a renowned physician, author and leading expert on healing, explains that trauma extends beyond the events that befall an individual.[48] Instead, it encompasses the profound internal impact that emerges from those experiences. Trauma represents a psychological wound that resides within a person. When triggered, this wound resurfaces with such force that it evokes the sensation of being struck again, as if for the very first time.

Maté distinguishes between two types of trauma wounds. The first is often rooted in abusive environments, encompassing sexual abuse, emotional abuse and other traumatic events. In the context of early childhood, trauma can stem from significant occurrences such as war, the loss of a parent, violence, addiction, separation or neglect. The second type of trauma emerges from unmet needs during childhood, such as the absence of unconditional love and acceptance, the burden of maintaining good relationships with parents, the longing for acceptance, and the repression of a wide range of emotions including anger, love and grief. The suppression of certain emotional experiences in a child, according to Maté, distorts their development and has implications for their future.

What also needs to be said is that an individual's response to a traumatic event is influenced by various factors, such as

---

48 Maté, G, Maté, D, *The Myth of Normal: Trauma, Illness, and Healing in a Toxic Culture*, Avery, 2022

their level of resilience, available support systems, and past experiences. While one person may perceive a physical attack as being not deeply traumatic, another may carry the wounds for years. Those with a history of trauma often exhibit distinct psychological and physical responses to stress. Additionally, the perception of future incidents is profoundly shaped by our worldview and self-image. If we view the world as dangerous and unpredictable, we are more likely to be deeply affected by traumatic events. Conversely, those who hold a different perspective may walk away from similar events with minimal impact. Each traumatic experience is deeply personal and unique to the individual.

When revisiting the past, it is essential to identify triggers and assess the coping strategies we have employed so far, to allow a deeper understanding of ourselves and our conditioning.

When we understand our triggers, reactions and behaviours, we can gain a better understanding of how to shift away from unhealthy patterns. This awareness allows us to determine which confidence-building tools to practise and which therapeutic approaches to choose, ensuring the safety of our psychological and physical wellbeing. By nurturing our internal strength, we reduce the likelihood of succumbing to adverse circumstances, and enhance our preparedness to effectively handle conflicts and potential physical threats.

Take Aways

- Trauma is a psychological wound that occurs in the aftermath of experiencing or witnessing a disturbing life event, or a series of disturbing events.
- Trauma can leave a person unable to cope, can cause a person to experience flashbacks, and can often lead to post-traumatic stress disorder (PTSD), which affects many women.
- Trauma affects each individual differently.

- Understanding trauma on an individual level is important, so that we can establish and put in place measures to protect ourselves from dangerous scenarios.

Coping Strategies: How Individuals Respond to Traumatic Events

To embark on the journey of healing from trauma, it is crucial to explore the coping mechanisms that we have, consciously or subconsciously, developed in order to shield ourselves from the overwhelming emotions associated with past traumatic experiences.

According to Sabina Sadecka, a systemic therapist and author, several coping strategies may be present:[49]

- **Exerting oneself:** This strategy involves engaging in activities that help us detach from the terrifying events unfolding around us, offering a temporary respite from the distress.
- **Being overly nice:** By adopting an excessively kind demeanour, we aim to protect ourselves from the aggression or harm that others may potentially inflict upon us.
- **Contracting the muscles:** Consciously tensing our muscles serves as a form of self-protection, creating a physical barrier against perceived threats.
- **Intellectualization:** This coping mechanism enables us to approach problems in a rational manner, focusing on logical analysis, while suppressing or avoiding the associated emotions.

These coping strategies act as stabilizing anchors that help shield us from perceived danger. They manifest as tendencies

---

49 Sadecka, S, "About Survival Strategies Without Which We Do Not Feel Safe", 2023, sabinasadecka.pl/o-strategiach-przetrwania-bez-ktorych-nie-czujemy-sie-bezpiecznie/

to overwork, to numb ourselves, or to disconnect from our authentic selves, providing temporary relief from the troubling feelings and emotions within us.

When our coping strategies are suddenly threatened, we may experience feelings of helplessness and being lost. Consequently, this can lead us to cling more tightly to our ways of coping – we may tense our muscles even harder, or work more intensely to desensitize ourselves to the emotional impact we are experiencing. If what previously shielded us from fear, intimidation and anger is no longer available for us to lean on, an overwhelming surge of emotions can surface, with an even greater impact. Several factors may contribute to the loss of our usual coping mechanisms, including the use of psychoactive substances that distort our sense of boundaries, receiving intense massages that release post-traumatic muscle tension, or engaging in practices such as yoga, breathing exercises, meditation and intense physical activity. Warm, non-judgemental and safe human contact can also unexpectedly weaken our psychological barriers, alleviating the need for constant self-protection, but also leaving us feeling utterly vulnerable.

Sadecka offers a captivating portrait of the interplay between protective tools and their connection to the healing process. The coping strategies we have cultivated can be visualized as bridges that span the gap between trauma and healing. Over time, these mechanisms can transform as we come to understand their purpose, gradually distancing ourselves from them in a caring and compassionate manner.

As we embark on our healing journeys, Sadecka's insights remind us of the transformative power we have within ourselves to bridge the gap between past trauma and a healthier future. Perhaps you, or someone you know, experienced a difficult childhood and has, as a result, developed a coping strategy of emotional detachment in order to shield themselves from further pain. This defence mechanism might have served as a bridge to tackle the challenging circumstances back then. However, over time, you may come to realize that this emotional detachment hinders the ability to form deep, meaningful connections with others and prevents you from experiencing true joy.

Being aware of the protective yet restrictive nature of these coping mechanisms can lead to a greater understanding of ourselves, enabling us to implement measures that will help us experience life in a more fulfilling way.

Likewise, if you have been a victim of past assault, the experience may have left you anxious and fearful. To break free from the protective mechanism of constant vigilance, you can begin working on methods that promote stability, balance and confidence. This chapter describes many such measures to help you determine and choose which ones may be helpful for you.

Take Aways

- Trauma-coping strategies can be both psychological and physical, including, for example, over-exerting ourselves, avoidance, or muscle tension.
- Coping strategies are bridges between healing and trauma. We can learn how to move away from them slowly, with compassion.

The Journey to Recovery

The term "healing" originates from an Old English word that means "wholeness". According to Dr Maté, when trauma disconnects us from our authentic inner selves, healing entails reconnecting with ourselves in order to achieve a state of wholeness. The journey toward wholeness becomes possible when we cultivate awareness in our lives and experiences.

For women who are healing from trauma, it is crucial to reflect on the factors ingrained in our female conditioning that have contributed to denying our wholeness. As we explored in Chapter 1: Women's Power, the "good girl" was taught to suppress anger, prioritize the needs of others over her own, and fulfil obligations and responsibilities, often at the expense of self-care. She aimed to avoid disappointing anyone and sought validation and acceptance. To break free from good girl conditioning, we discussed strategies such as asserting oneself in a verbal exchange and establishing personal boundaries. Maté also suggests that an effective tool for moving toward wholeness and healing is learning to say no more assertively.[50]

Overcoming Good Girl Conditioning: Challenging Societal Expectations

The good girl often struggles to say no, but is this ingrained in her nature? Probably not.

As Dr Maté explains, it is natural for children to say no frequently as part of their early programming, which allows them to develop into independent individuals with a sense of their own wishes, desires and values. Saying no helps children cultivate independence.

When we lose the ability to say no, we also lose a sense of our personal boundaries. When we wish to reject something and fail to do so, this can lead to resentment and physical effects on our bodies. It becomes a complex, stressful and exhausting cycle. We find ourselves trapped, communicating indirectly to avoid inflicting pain, trying to please everyone; all the while our self-protective mechanisms come crumbling down.

Many of us have experienced the denial of authenticity in the past, preventing us from staying true to ourselves, and in turn compromising our survival mechanisms. The feelings that served as valuable indicators, guiding us and notifying us

---

50 Maté, G, Maté, D, *The Myth of Normal: Trauma, Illness, and Healing in a Toxic Culture*, Avery, 2022

of important matters, were disregarded. We were unable to express ourselves freely, fearing that it would jeopardize our attachment to our caregivers. As a result, we suppressed our authenticity to such an extent that we dishonoured messages from our environment. Our gut feelings became obsolete.

Have you ever experienced this disconnect within yourself? You may have neglected your own values, or continuously put other people's needs before your own, and this could have occurred in your workplace, in your relationship, or at home with your family. Perhaps you've noticed that you are overly polite and people-pleasing, and this is starting to have a knock-on effect on your psychological or physical health. To determine whether this is the case for you in the present, pay close attention to your emotional reactions in certain situations. If you experience internal suffering or the feeling of shame, it is likely a sign of self-betrayal – you may be consciously or unconsciously doing something against your will, or compromising your values.

If we continuously misalign with our true selves, causing emotional distress or evoking negative emotions, with time our bodies will send us signals of illness. Such physical symptoms influenced by psychological or emotional factors are often referred to as psychosomatic signals, and can come in the form of headaches, stomach issues, skin conditions such as eczema, unexplained body pain, itching, or fatigue without apparent medical cause. Over time, we can become anxious or depressed.

By observing and analysing our patterns and body reactions, we can become aware of the conditioning that may be influencing us. Each experience can hold a lesson for us if we are willing to look within. During each difficult interaction, we can attempt to seek out the root cause of our triggers. Actively ask yourself: "Where does it come from?"

According to Dr Hans Selye, a prominent researcher in the area of stress, a significant portion of our stress arises from an intense urge to portray a persona that does not align with our true selves. Selye suggests that such inauthenticity, while being a major source of stress, actually serves as an adaptive response stemming from our early developmental experiences.[51]

You may be wondering what all of this has to do with healing trauma, so let's take a moment to think about it. If your traumatic experience from childhood involved resisting your true authentic self, the mechanisms you developed as a result may have created wounds that reopen whenever you get triggered. To avoid these triggers, you need to start setting boundaries, as discussed within the context of the good girl conditioning.

To recap, healing will occur when you:

- Learn how to say no
- Find healthy ways to express anger
- Stop prioritizing others' needs at the expense of your own health and wellbeing
- Break free from the constant need to be overly nice and pleasing others.

When you say no and experience the sense of a weight being lifted, followed by a sense of relief, this may be a sign that you have just released the grip of good girl conditioning. Similarly, when you assert yourself while protecting your boundaries, you will start to feel a sense of calm and peace, alongside an inner feeling of self-respect.

The confidence-building tools described in earlier chapters, such as mindfulness and effective communication, will help you cultivate self-awareness and assertiveness. By shifting the dynamic from the repressed emotions of the good girl to the empowered version of your true self, you can start to fully express who you are. You can practise these strategies on your own, by seeking support from trusted friends, or by consulting with a specialist in the field.

---

51 Selye, H, *The Stress of Life*, McGraw-Hill Education, 1978

Tapping into Your True Authentic Self

During the journey of trauma healing and the exploration of our true authentic selves, there are specific strategies that can aid in the discovery of our inner nature. Some of these strategies have been previously discussed, including setting boundaries, which entails listening to our needs and effectively communicating them to others. In conjunction with boundary assertion, it is essential to identify our core values. When we align our actions and behaviours with these values, we become more authentic and true to ourselves. Additionally, engaging in practices of mindfulness and compassion cultivates greater awareness, and fosters a deeper understanding of our own nature.

Another significant approach to tapping into our inner spirit is through self-reflection. This involves exploring our thoughts and feelings through activities such as journaling or meditation. Various forms of therapy can also help to facilitate this introspective process.

Along the path of uncovering our true inner selves, it is valuable to reconnect with our passions and hobbies, or to explore new avenues that bring fulfilment to our daily lives. Engaging in activities that ignite passion and joy allow us to reconnect with our authentic selves. Furthermore, this journey may involve forging connections with others, whether it be reconnecting with old friends or fostering new friendships.

The Power of Support and Social Connection in Healing

Do you remember walking down the street, with neighbours regularly stopping you for a chat, or when a friend paid you a surprise visit by unexpectedly knocking on your door?

If you fall into the category of Generation X or Millennials, you are likely to recall the days, before the internet, when human interaction relied largely on physical proximity to other people and you engaged with others without the use of cell phones or social media.

With the emergence of fascinating technological tools, we have become more digitally linked, but much less attached in the physical world. The tools that were intended to bring us closer together, have, ironically, led us to a greater social disconnection than humans have ever experienced before. With depression, anxiety and death by suicide on the rise, we find ourselves descending further into the rabbit hole of separation.

If we delve deeper into the past, we notice a significant shift in the way that we, as humans, live. We have strayed away from living in communities – securely maintained environments – where children had multiple adult and parental figures. Today, families often find themselves isolated from extended relatives, with limited attachment. We learn to live independently and in solitude. This type of disconnection and isolation leads us further toward separation and, ultimately, into a variety of stress responses, as explained by Dr Gabor Maté.[52]

We don't have to look far to find proof of how this social phenomenon is linked to our wellbeing. Studies have demonstrated that social connectedness protects adults in the general population from depressive symptoms and disorders.[53] On the other side of the spectrum, one profound study showed that social isolation had effects that were the same as smoking 15 cigarettes a day, and also had more detrimental health effects than suffering from high blood pressure and obesity.[54] The same study showed

---

52 Maté, G, Maté, D, *The Myth of Normal: Trauma, Illness, and Healing in a Toxic Culture*, Avery, 2022

53 Wickramaratne, PJ, et al., "Social Connectedness as a Determinant of Mental Health: A Scoping Review", *PloS one*, vol. 17(10), 2022, e0275004, doi.org/10.1371/journal.pone.0275004

54 Holt-Lunstad, J, et al., "Social Relationships and Mortality Risk: A Meta-analytic Review", *PLoS medicine*, vol. 7(7), 2010, e1000316, doi.org/10.1371/journal.pmed.1000316

that those with stronger social connections had a reduced mortality risk compared to those with weaker social links. Furthermore, people who are more attached to others have better self-esteem, greater empathy and are more trusting and cooperative. Feeling connected to others promotes emotional and physical wellbeing, which is paramount on the journey of healing and growth.

Community support is beneficial for everyone, including those struggling with good girl conditioning, and those who have experienced violence and abuse. Social networks can play a vital role in helping to restore our inner strength and achieve a sense of balance and stability. If you find it challenging to receive support from family members or work colleagues, it may be helpful to explore joining specialized meet-up groups, taking up new hobbies, or actively participating in local community projects.

Perhaps it is also time to acknowledge that sharing our stories and asking for help can be beneficial. It can begin by opening up to a compassionate friend who can relate to your experience, or by forging new social connections. Whichever path you choose, finding your tribe can have a significant positive impact on your healing journey.

Take Aways

- To facilitate healing from trauma, it is crucial to acknowledge the coping strategies we have utilized so far, and to gradually distance ourselves from potentially detrimental habits.
- It is important to become aware of our past conditioning, so that we are able to begin asserting our personal boundaries and to practise assertiveness.
- By connecting with others, we can become more self-assured and foster the feeling of community and support, contributing to our overall wellbeing.

Therapies for Trauma

The treatment of trauma varies across the world, and is influenced by factors such as cultural beliefs, available resources and healthcare systems. Common methods include psychotherapy, pharmacology (medications), group therapy, self-care, and complementary (alternative) approaches. The accessibility of these interventions varies by location and it is important to seek treatment approaches that are adapted culturally.

When deciding on the best form of therapy, it is crucial to identify and acknowledge personal needs and preferences in order to determine the most suitable method. Conducting research and establishing trust with a specialized professional in a one-on-one or group setting can greatly aid the process. In cases where local resources are limited or unavailable, online support for trauma treatment can also be valuable.

In this chapter we will go through some of the mainstream approaches for the treatment of trauma, as well as other integrative methodologies.

Cognitive Behavioural Therapy (CBT)
Cognitive Behavioural Therapy remains one of the most common therapies for the treatment of trauma. Its aim is to assist trauma survivors in learning to identify the patterns of thinking and behaviour that contribute to the maintenance of trauma symptoms. CBT typically involves several components, including cognitive restructuring, situational and imagery exposure, psychoeducation, and anxiety management techniques, such as breathing and relaxation training. In cognitive restructuring, the focus is on identifying unhelpful negative thought patterns and replacing them with realistic, balanced and positive alternative perspectives. Exposure therapy gradually exposes trauma survivors to their traumatic memories in a safe environment. This can be achieved through activities such as recounting the traumatic

event. Over time, this exposure helps to reduce distress and fear associated with the traumatic experience. The psychoeducational component of CBT equips individuals with strategies to manage trauma-related symptoms. These skills may include stress management, problem solving, communication skills and relaxation exercises.

By combining knowledge with practical solutions, participants gain a sense of control over the healing process and acquire strategies that can be applied in their daily lives outside of therapy sessions.

CBT also involves the creation of a safety plan for trauma survivors. This includes identifying triggers and implementing self-care strategies. Building a supportive network and adopting coping mechanisms for stress management are integral parts of this safety planning process. These measures empower individuals to effectively manage trauma symptoms and regain a sense of control.

CBT methods, to an extent, can be practised by an individual through education in the form of self-help books, online resources and apps that can help you go through CBT exercises and interventions. Many of those will include journaling, recognizing negative thought patterns, setting realistic goals, relaxation techniques, and developing coping strategies.

Eye Movement Desensitization and Reprocessing (EMDR)

Eye Movement Desensitization and Reprocessing is a structured therapy, widely used in the US and the UK, that focuses on traumatic memories and how they are stored in the brain. During EMDR sessions, patients briefly concentrate on the traumatic memory while experiencing bilateral stimulation, typically through eye movement. Bilateral stimulation engages both sides of the brain by moving the body in a rhythmic fashion.

The goal of this stimulation is to reduce the vividness and emotional intensity associated with the memory.

EMDR is specifically designed for the treatment of trauma and its effects, including anxiety and depression. The therapy aims to reprocess traumatic memories, gradually desensitizing the distressing aspects over time through repeated EMDR sessions. By integrating traumatic experiences into the past, individuals can reduce the emotional disturbance associated with these events in their everyday lives.

Cognitive Processing Therapy (CPT)
Cognitive Processing Therapy is a specific form of Cognitive Behavioural Therapy, designed to address and modify unhelpful beliefs related to trauma. It is effective in reducing symptoms of post-traumatic stress associated with traumatic events such as abuse and rape. CPT focuses on the strong connection between thoughts and emotions, aiming to help patients understand how traumatic events have influenced their beliefs about themselves and the world. The therapy method assists individuals in breaking down patterns of thoughts and feelings associated with trauma, ultimately leading to the transformation of maladaptive thought processes. Through CPT, patients can regain a sense of trust and control that may have been lost as a result of their traumatic experiences.

While working with a trained specialist is recommended, self-practice of CPT may also be helpful. This would include educating yourself through resources such as self-help books, online materials and worksheets.

Dialectal Behaviour Therapy (DBT)
Dialectical Behaviour Therapy is a modified form of Cognitive Behavioural Therapy that aims to help individuals develop healthy coping mechanisms for stress and emotional regulation. It has also been found effective in the treatment of post-traumatic stress disorder.

Within DBT, there are two techniques used to address extreme emotions: "opposite action" and "all the way opposite action". The underlying principle of these techniques is that if our emotions correspond to reality, we are encouraged to act on them. However, if our emotions do not align with reality, we are instructed to act in the opposite way.[55]

To provide an example in the context of experiencing fear, it is important to determine whether our feelings are associated with actual danger, and whether or not environmental cues indicate a genuine threat. If there is no real danger present, we can engage in opposite action by disregarding the behavioural urge to flee or to avoid facing our fears.

A great example of this at play is getting on a bus. If we experience fear that causes us to feel frozen and unmotivated to act (ie, a fear of getting on a bus), we need to exert a level of self-command to do the opposite of what the fear is dictating – in this case, we need to tell ourselves to get on the bus even though we are scared, because there is no genuine threat to our safety by getting on a bus. In that moment, employing self-talk can be helpful, as we programme ourselves to confront and overcome our fears. In similar situations, when we feel threatened and tempted to freeze with no escape route in sight, we must find inner strength to break free from our fear and command ourselves to take action.

In the "all the way opposite action", a person who experiences social anxiety and who therefore avoids social situations, would deliberately seek out human interaction and take active part in social gatherings. With consistent practice of this type of opposite action, the person will gradually learn how their fear and anxiety are not as threatening as previously believed. In this way, an individual can build coping skills, and find new confidence and a sense of control.

To help you picture the extreme opposite action, I'll tell you a story that was told to me. During a colleague's childhood, there was a local stalker and exhibitionist who

---

55 Velikova, K (clinical psychologist), 2023, personal interview

used to startle women by jumping out of various hiding places, exposing himself in a shocking manner. One day, this individual targeted a female, who, instead of reacting in fear and distress, shouted out a big joyful, "Yes!" upon his approach. This unexpected response completely caught the man off guard, and he quickly retreated in total shock.

By practising these types of opposite action approaches, we can challenge and face our fears. In that sense, DBT therapy empowers individuals to confront and effectively manage their emotions, promoting personal growth and wellbeing.

Cognitive Analytic Therapy (CAT)

Cognitive Analytic Therapy can be helpful for trauma victims who have identified with the victim role and in turn have developed negative beliefs about themselves and the world. With negative, distorted and detrimental views, a person can identify with and engage in behaviours that will further reinforce their beliefs, perpetuating a cycle of victimization. The triggers will keep resurfacing over time, until we become aware of this conditioning and tackle the problem at its core.

The mere act of being aware of and identifying our conditioning may not be enough. It is crucial to train ourselves how to respond appropriately to trauma or attacks, creating new automatic responses. By practising how to embody a different role, we can shift into the mindset of an attacker, or an active defender. With this approach, CAT offers a valuable form of treatment for trauma, challenging a person's identification with the victim role, helping to develop healthier responses to traumatic experiences.

If this form of therapy is unavailable to you, investigate different resources about CAT to gain a wider understanding of this approach. CAT uses a variety of different tools and worksheets for the exploration of patterns of thinking, and for identifying recurring patterns in relationships. You can find some of these tools online or in books, and these can help guide you through the process of self-exploration.

Take Aways

- Various trauma treatment approaches are available through wider health systems, including Cognitive Behavioural Therapy, Eye Movement Desensitization and Reprocessing, Cognitive Processing Therapy, Dialectal Behaviour Therapy and Cognitive Analytic Therapy.
- Approaches to therapy should be treated individually, and specialist treatment that has been culturally adapted should be sought out.

Ancient Voices in the Present: Exploring Integrative Therapies

Introduction to Integrative Therapies

Throughout history, many different cultures have recognized the interconnectedness of the body and mind in healing and promoting wellbeing. Examples of such practices include acupuncture, qigong and yoga. In Indigenous cultures around the world, we can track traditional healing practices that encompass rituals, dances and bodywork aimed at restoring balance and facilitating the release of emotional ailments. While ancient practices may not always directly align with modern bodywork therapies, they share a common focus on integrating the body, mind and spirit to achieve healing and create a sense of equilibrium.

Integrative therapies, sometimes considered as complementary or alternative medicine, encompass a wide range of practices and approaches. They can be used as standalone practices, or alongside and in conjunction with "conventional" treatments.

Integrative therapies seek to establish equilibrium in the mind, the body and the spirit, striving for a holistic understanding of the individual. They harness the body's innate healing abilities while nurturing a high quality of life. These therapies embrace the notion that a fulfilled existence encompasses not only freedom from disease, but also the cultivation of purpose and vitality.

Some integrative therapies include:

- **Acupuncture:** An ancient practice involving the use of needles targeted on specific points of the human body to stimulate energy flow and to restore balance
- **Herbal medicine:** The use of herbs and plants to promote healing
- **Massage therapy:** Manual manipulation of the body's soft tissues, promoting circulation, reducing muscle tension and soreness, and inducing relaxation
- **Mind-body techniques:** Practices such as meditation, yoga, mindfulness, tai chi, etc, aimed at reducing stress, improving awareness and enhancing overall health
- **Chiropractic treatment:** Aligning the musculoskeletal system, with special attention to spinal alignment, to promote mobility and alleviate pain and tension in the body
- **Homeopathy:** The use of substances that stimulate the body's natural ability to heal and restore equilibrium
- **Naturopathy:** Encompassing various approaches, including diet and nutrition, herbal remedies, lifestyle changes and other treatments
- **Energy therapies:** Therapies such as reiki and qigong, which aim to restore the body's energy fields and promote healing.

Before engaging in any of these practices, please ensure that you conduct your own research, or consult with a health professional, in order to choose the most appropriate treatment and service provider for your individual needs.

Somatic Therapies: Connecting with the Body

Somatic therapies, also known as body-centred therapies, focus on the physical sensations experienced in the body to facilitate healing. They employ techniques such as breath work and movement to assist in releasing tension associated with trauma, and to reduce stress stored within the body. Somatic therapies can be used alongside counselling or talk therapy.

Somatic therapies can help individuals improve their patterns of thought and rewire their brains to focus on body sensations and control of the emotional system. Somatic therapies can improve body awareness and can help to create a conscious connection between body and mind. This form of therapy can support individuals in overcoming psychological, emotional and physical barriers that stand in the way of improving mental health.

Proponents of somatic therapies suggest that by reconnecting with the body to release trauma, the symptoms of PTSD can become more manageable. Additionally, somatic therapies also aim to alleviate physical tension, addressing emotional dysregulation and freezing, which can be crucial when establishing a sense of self-control.

Somatic Experiencing Therapy: Healing Trauma through Body Awareness

Dr Peter Levine, a psychotherapist and creator of the Somatic Experiencing methodology, took inspiration from nature for this treatment approach, after observing the animal kingdom. Levine noticed that animals who are often in danger manage to quickly recuperate by trembling and shaking to release their stress energy. His method aims to connect body and mind, to help people identify the areas of tension in their bodies which occur as a result of past traumatic experiences.[56]

According to Levine, flashbacks and heightened awareness states, among many other side-effects of trauma, are caused by changes and disturbances in the autonomic nervous

---

56 https://www.somaticexperiencing.com/somatic-experiencing

system. His approach is to provide the autonomic nervous system with the tools needed to self-regulate. In this type of therapy treatment, clients become more aware of their emotions and their bodily reactions to stress. They observe where and how the stress is stored in their bodies.

Various studies have shown promising results for Somatic Experiencing therapy's treatment of PTSD symptoms and anxiety, as the therapy was reported to improve emotional regulation and overall wellbeing. One study revealed that after Somatic Experiencing treatment, 44 per cent of participants were no longer diagnosed with PTSD.[57]

Osho's Dynamic Meditation: Combining Movement and Mindfulness

Osho's dynamic meditation may take you back to tribal times, as the practice often resembles wild dances, accompanied by drums and chanting. This powerful meditation method was developed by an Indian spiritual teacher, Osho, with the aim of helping individuals to release energy blocks stored within the body, including pent-up emotions and mental tensions.

By engaging in intense breath work and movement, the practice allows for a release of repressed emotions. The underlying principle is to facilitate a free flow of energy, removing any blockages stored in the body.

The practice consists of several stages, each serving a different purpose. It begins with rapid breathing to oxygenate the body, followed by catharsis, which involves the release of emotions through unrepressed physical movement and vocalization. This is followed by vigorous jumping, and later, a stage of stillness, where participants remain motionless in silence, and finally, a phase of celebration expressed through joyful dance.

57 Brom, D, et al., "Somatic Experiencing for Posttraumatic Stress Disorder: A Randomized Controlled Outcome Study", *Journal of Traumatic Stress*, vol. 30(3), 2017, pp. 304–12. doi:10.1002/jts.22189

In my personal experience of dynamic meditation, I found I was able to significantly reduce my levels of stress and allow for an uninhibited release of stored-up emotions, which emerged during some of the stages of the meditation. The practice allowed for an integration of repressed feelings, with a comforting and compassionate soothing phase. It allowed me to transcend the conscious mind and enter a deeper state of relaxation, freedom of self-expression, and gratitude.

If you are not ready to take part in a group session to practise this form of meditation, there are online video tutorials which you can follow at home to discover the benefits of this method.

Ecstatic Dance: Expressive Movement for Emotional Release

Ecstatic dance is a form of movement which encourages people to experience self-discovery, promotes emotional release, and seeks connection between the body and the present moment.

The dance encourages the feeling of joy and liberation, allowing participants a chance to immerse themselves in creative self-expression. For many, it is a form of meditation that allows for a deeper alignment with the self, and with a community of fellow dancers.

For me personally, ecstatic dance is a chance to express myself freely and intuitively, without judgement. It also allows a fascinating observation of how others involved in the practice manage to peel away their self-protective layers of security to allow for a deeper connection within themselves through movement.

Similar to other forms of meditation, you can follow this type of practice at home, as a range of online videos are available on the internet.

Meditation: Cultivating Mindfulness and Inner Peace

Meditation can encompass any form of training that focuses the mind. It can help bring about mental clarity, a state of calmness, and inner stillness. In most forms of meditation, the attention is directed inward, often by focusing on a particular thought or item, or even on a particular activity. It can also be the cultivation of mindfulness through non-judgemental awareness.

Meditation can be one of the most calming tools for the treatment of trauma, helping individuals to gain a state of relaxation and stillness. Some of the meditation approaches worth mentioning include:

Mindfulness-Based Stress Reduction (MBSR) combines mindfulness meditation with body movements and the practice of body awareness. For trauma survivors, it is especially helpful in order to develop better awareness, and to aid in regulating emotions. The practice can also prove helpful in cultivating self-compassion, which is used in various trauma-related interventions.

Trauma Sensitive Yoga incorporates movement (postures), breath work and mindfulness. One important study, which ran between 2008 and 2011, led by Bessel van der Kolk and a team from the Trauma Center at the Justice Resource Institute, examined the effectiveness of this method for women with chronic PTSD. It was found that the group studying yoga (when compared to the group who received a health education intervention instead) had significantly reduced symptoms of PTSD, depression and anxiety, and their sleep quality had improved.[58]

---

58 van der Kolk, B A, et al., "Yoga as an Adjunctive Treatment for Posttraumatic Stress Disorder: A Randomized Controlled Trial", *Journal of Clinical Psychiatry*, vol. 75(6), 2014, pp. e559–65. doi:10.4088/JCP.13m08561

Yoga Nidra can be a helpful technique for healing from trauma, as it guides individuals to enter a state of deep relaxation and rest. Yoga nidra allows for increased body awareness, which can promote healing and create a sense of safety and stability. Through various visualizations in the practice, individuals can learn to cultivate qualities such as self-compassion and resilience. The practice helps to integrate all aspects of the self by creating space for acceptance, allowing emotions to be processed in a safe and relaxed environment.

Loving-Kindness Meditation is a very soothing practice of forming kind intentions toward yourself and the world. In this space, trauma victims can cultivate self-compassion, and evoke positive emotions to promote healing.

Body Scan Meditation is a form of meditation that directs a participant's attention to various parts of the body in order to promote relaxation and awareness. It can be beneficial for the treatment of trauma, as this practice is deeply connected to the body. Participants observe and then release any areas of tension.

Breath Awareness Meditation is a common technique for relaxation, especially among trauma survivors. It focuses on grounding the individual and helping them regulate their emotions through focusing on their breath. With the attention focused inward on the breath and its qualities, people can experience a reduction of stress and anxiety, which can also be beneficial for those who experience stress-related triggers and hypervigilance.

Guided Imagery, also known as guided visualization or mental imagery, is a type of relaxation meditation, where participants focus on concentrating on a specific object, sound or experience. Its goal is to help people achieve a state of calmness. During guided imagery, we often visualize a peaceful place, or a peaceful scenario. In this practice we are guided by a facilitator, or an audio recording, to enter a state in which we focus on images and sensory details to create vivid pictures, with our eyes closed. We usually go into a pleasant, calming scenario, imagining ourselves in a soothing environment, usually involving nature. Connecting to all senses, we can immerse ourselves in a peaceful and tranquil environment which evokes positive emotions, and creates a sense of ease and peacefulness.

* * *

When practising meditation for the first time, it is helpful to use **guided meditation** such as the guided imagery mentioned previously, or guided breathing, body scans, muscle relaxation, or various types of visualization. This can be done by going to a class and listening to a facilitator, or by listening to a recording that will guide you through the experience.

Take Aways

- Various meditative practices can be helpful in reducing stress and anxiety and in promoting a state of calmness. These practices can be used as part of an ongoing stress-relief-related therapy approach, or a stand-alone practice for those who don't require other forms of therapy intervention.
- If you find it difficult to practise by yourself, find a facilitator, or a recording that can guide you through the meditative process.

EXERCISE: GROUNDING MEDITATION

In the following exercise, I present an example of a **grounding meditation,** which can be used as a relaxation tool, and, when recovering from trauma, as a technique for stress reduction and anxiety management.

- Find a comfortable seat, either lying down or assuming a position in which you are able to remain relaxed while in a state of awareness.
- Acknowledge your breath. Start taking deep inbreaths, inhaling through the nose and exhaling either through the nose, or through the mouth.
- Pay close attention to the sensations of your breath entering and leaving your body. Scan your body for any physical sensations, such as tension or relaxation.
- Focus on the area beneath you and the connection of your body to the surface on which you are resting.
- Envision the space beneath you as a supportive foundation, carrying your weight. Imagine roots extending directly from your feet (when standing) or from your tailbone (when seated), penetrating the ground and creating a connection between you and the Earth or the surface beneath you. Picture these roots growing and strengthening, firmly anchoring you to the ground.
- Involve your senses, noticing sounds around you, the temperature of your body and the surrounding environment. Recognize any smells present. Engage your senses as much as you can, remaining connected to what they feel like in the present moment.
- Use self-talk to reaffirm your sensations, saying things such as, "I feel grounded, I feel supported", or "I am connected in the here and now".

- If your mind starts to wander, without judgement, bring your attention back to your breath and to your body.
- When you're ready to close this practice, gently bring your attention back to the natural rhythm of your breath and your surroundings, gently opening your eyes.

Martial Arts: Finding Empowerment and Resilience

We have previously discussed how physical activity and training can act as a tool in trauma prevention, and how it can prepare us for conflicts and threats. We mentioned how it can serve as a great confidence booster, counteracting the feelings of helplessness and anger that are often associated with PTSD.

In my personal and professional opinion, among the diverse range of training options available, self-defence and martial arts offer exceptionally strong foundations for rebuilding yourself after experiencing trauma. Over the past 20 years, I have witnessed remarkable transformations in various communities, particularly among vulnerable groups such as children, female adolescents, women and minority populations, as they embrace the empowering practice of arts such as Brazilian jiu-jitsu. To illustrate this, I would like to share the story of a woman who, as a survivor of sexual assault, utilized martial arts training as a pathway to reclaim her power.

Syriah, from Colorado, turned to Brazilian jiu-jitsu as a means of gaining confidence after serving in the military for ten years. When she first set foot on the training mat, her primary concern was her security and self-assurance. However, Syriah quickly discovered that her journey in the martial art transformed her from an angry and reserved individual Into a self-driven, motivated and composed person. The skills she acquired through practising jiu-jitsu opened up numerous opportunities in her professional life.

Syriah, who battles chronic post-traumatic stress disorder resulting from a past assault, wholeheartedly affirms that practising martial arts has been instrumental in her journey of coping with the condition. Finding solace in the jiu-jitsu community, she discovered a sanctuary where she could release her frustrations and channel her energy positively. The demanding training regimen not only impressed upon her the significance of mindfulness, but also taught her the art of living in the present moment. Syriah firmly believes that embarking on this transformative journey has unequivocally been the greatest decision she has ever made for herself.

For Syriah, training in Jiu-jitsu required facing her fears and meeting challenges head-on, throwing herself into a form of prolonged exposure therapy. She reflected on how jiu-jitsu initially served as a catalyst for opening up and expressing emotions, as training sometimes evoked tears, which is often the case with trauma survivors. However, Syriah found comfort in the encouraging and understanding jiu-jitsu community – her fellow training partners would help her during vulnerable moments, offering unwavering support.

While not every person is immediately ready or able to push themselves into a group martial arts training routine to rebuild their inner strength, there are various practice approaches that we can seek to aid the recovery process. The journey can start by getting involved with a female personal trainer, or by training with a trusted friend.

The act of practising defensive techniques can increase your confidence, and help you to establish a sense of control over your safety. Various forms of training can also provide a means for releasing tension that is stored in the body, allowing for emotional and physical catharsis. By integrating the body–mind connection, the consistent practice of martial arts will enhance the awareness of your body, and help you to remain focused. This reconnection between body and mind can also be grounding and promote a greater sense of presence, which is important for trauma survivors.

For those whose self-confidence has been eroded by traumatic experiences, martial arts offer new opportunities for growth and the achievement of goals. These specific training practices can build a sense of self-worth, self-esteem and inner strength.

In a supportive training environment, the initial feeling of discomfort through exposure, close physical contact and potential pressure to the body will be comforted by the release of mood-boosting hormones and by positive feedback from coaches and fellow practitioners.

As you go through physical scenarios where you are being held or pinned, your body learns how to react appropriately in dealing with stress, pressure and discomfort. You become accustomed to the feelings, as your body recognizes these as training practices, rather than threats, which can lead to rebuilding healthy connections with other people, both physically and psychologically.

Lastly, another crucial aspect of martial arts and self-defence training is the unparalleled bond within the community. It fosters a profound sense of belonging, empathy and camaraderie. For trauma survivors, this robust support system proves invaluable, as fellow practitioners offer steadfast encouragement and dedicated assistance. These aspects serve as powerful catalysts in the transformative journey of healing.

Take Aways

- Alternative and integrative therapies that focus on the mind–body connection can help in releasing the remnants of trauma that are stored in the body.

- Somatic methods that involve body movements allow for a deeper sense of connection to the self, and provide a more holistic approach to healing.
- Certain methods such as Somatic Experiencing therapy or trauma sensitive yoga, together with holistic approaches such as Osho's dynamic meditation, ecstatic dancing and meditation offer alternative routes toward healing.
- Martial arts and self-defence offer a multifaceted approach to healing from trauma, encompassing empowerment, emotional release, self-esteem enhancement, stress relief and a supportive community.

Neuroplasticity: Unlocking the Potential for Healing and Growth

Alongside our understanding about how best to increase confidence and address trauma (as explained throughout this book – eg, physical activity, meditation, CBT and other therapies, and so on), there is also one other crucial aspect to consider: scientific reassurance that change is accessible to all of us through the brain's neuroplasticity – the brain's ability to form new neural pathways.

In the past, it was widely believed that our brains were hardwired by the time we reached our early twenties. However, recent discoveries have shown that our brains continue to grow and reorganize themselves beyond this age. They possess the remarkable capacity to rewire and adapt by remapping previously received information. New thought processes, behaviours and habits have the potential to reshape the brain's structure. The more neural connections we create, the weaker the old patterns become. Although the time required for this process varies from person to person, ranging from weeks or months to years in some cases, positive reframing and rewiring are reliable paths toward progress and growth.

Each deliberate action taken to cultivate these transformative habits contributes not only to our overall wellbeing, but also equips us with invaluable confidence tools on our journey of healing from trauma. Rest assured, science's understanding smiles upon us, showing us that a path away from the old and a gateway toward the new does indeed exist. Regardless of the length of the process, profound change remains well within our reach.

Various forms of therapy described in this chapter, as well as self-help tools, can guide you toward the healing process. On the way to recovering from violence-related trauma, choose the methods carefully, ideally consulting with professionals in the field. The more you explore, the more you may find that some approaches work better than others, or are better suited to your individual needs and experiences.

Take Aways

- Science confirms that we can reshape our brain, forming new neural connections by changing our thought patterns, behaviours and habits.
- The scientific research is reassuring for those suffering from trauma and mental health conditions, as it gives hope that we have the capacity within our minds to effect positive change.
- Choose the professionals you want to work with carefully, and explore various healing methods for violence-related trauma that may suit your needs.

Conclusion

The wisdom needed to build, learn and heal is within our reach, inside each one of us. While pain and suffering are inevitable and inseparable parts of our human experience, it is within the presence of suffering, not in the absence of it, that we can grow. On the path to reclaiming our confidence, and recovering from traumatic experiences, we need to consider and acknowledge our whole entire being.

We can start by mindfully looking inside of ourselves for signs of unhealthy programming, such as good girl conditioning, and other social boundaries that we feel we must conform to. As we uncover the thought patterns and behaviours that no longer serve us, it is crucial that we establish healthy habits, and learn how to develop and employ strong verbal and non-verbal strategies, including good communication skills. With exploration of techniques such as role play and positive self-talk, we can further improve our assertiveness and build resilience. Adding breath work practice to our confidence toolbox can also help expand our awareness, allowing us to regulate emotionally, enhancing our capacity to cope, and improving our overall quality of life. Incorporating all of these empowerment tools will not only be paramount to our safety for in-the-moment support, but it will also contribute to our personal growth.

*　*　*

When it comes to recovering from trauma, it is beneficial to recognize the triggers, evaluate the coping mechanisms we have employed so far, and consider seeking professional treatment methods when needed. Above all, as advised by Dr Gabor Maté, it is essential to reconnect with our authentic inner self.[59]

Seeking the answers within is the start of any successful heroine's journey. As we venture along the path of facing the demons of trauma, and slaying the dragons of fear, we reconnect with our inner strengths on the way to achieving wholeness.

---

59 Maté, G, Maté, D, *The Myth of Normal: Trauma, Illness, and Healing in a Toxic Culture*, Avery, 2022

I invite you to contemplate our modern capitalistic pursuits, which often foster greater separateness and loneliness, and to reflect upon our true human nature, reminding ourselves that collaboration is, in fact, our biggest innate purpose. Building and nurturing social connections will serve as steadfast pillars of support throughout our healing journey. By working together, we can conquer the challenges of isolation and rediscover the transformative power of community in nurturing our wellbeing and resilience.

Taking a significant stride toward cultivating a healthier and more conscious society should involve introducing trauma awareness and stress education in schools. This pivotal step would allow us to recognize and embrace each other's unique qualities, forming stronger connections and promoting greater understanding of one another.

As we embark on our trauma-healing journeys, we are fortunate to have a range of treatment approaches available to us. Whichever method(s) you choose, remember that support is always within reach, whether in the form of professional therapy offered by your local health service, through your social network, or even online. The initial step is learning how to ask for help and being prepared to embark on a transformative journey of self-discovery, where the rebirth of confidence and empowerment will take place. Countless individuals have walked this path before you, and you can do it too. There lies a power within you, waiting to rebuild and reshape you into the strong, resilient female warrior.

CONCLUSION

When we talk about women's safety in the 21st century, and how this applies to the western world, it's essential to take a closer look at the intricate social dynamics and the common narratives that surround us. We need to cast a discerning eye over the ways in which we are brought up, and how our cultures shape our everyday lives. It's important to recognize the areas in which we may be compromising our boundaries, suffocating the intuitive inner voices, and putting our safety at risk.

Understanding that most threats against women are perpetrated by non-strangers and that younger females are the most vulnerable group likely to face sexual violence and coercion, we should expand our approach to self-defence. This means considering a broader range of behavioural, psychological and physical tools to improve our safety.

* * *

The initial step toward becoming an empowered female is to observe our conditioning, the signals we convey through our unique body language, and the way we express ourselves.

We can learn how to improve our verbal and non-verbal communication, and start to employ various strategies, both as preventative measures (conflict resolution), and for boundary assertion (protecting our safety).

We can further empower ourselves in the physical dojo, with a variety of different training methods available. These practices can condition the body, and improve our strength and our reaction time. The skills we gain from physical practice will also translate into a more confident mindset, and help prevent extreme traumatization.

It's worth remembering that both mental and physical preparation are crucial, especially during moments when our nervous system triggers the "fight or flight" response, and in the presence of imminent physical threats. Preventative measures and preparing ourselves to face the unexpected remains one of the best methods to practise self-defence.

* * *

As you start to explore the self-defence empowerment tactics and techniques, it's important to keep in mind that stepping out of your comfort zone is rarely easy. Handling conflicts and taking on physical challenges can feel daunting, and it takes time and practice to become more confident in our actions. However, these are the skills worth spending a lifetime building. The confidence tools you use, and the effort you put in, may be the turning point in how you show up in the world, especially during times that threaten your safety.

Every time you stand up for yourself, you reinforce the idea that you are powerful. One day, you will suddenly realize that you embody the qualities of the female warrior you have been wanting to become. You will listen to her certainty and wisdom, her inner voice of intuition, staying assured in your skills and abilities. And when the time comes, you will stay strong, ready to fight back.

* * *

When we examine the statistical data of assaults against women, it begs for a deeper enquiry into the lives of females, particularly the younger generation. It also forces us to contemplate the various factors that contribute to susceptibility to grooming and manipulation.

It's time to change the narrative and begin teaching young women that their opinions matter, their dreams and desires are valuable, and that they have the right to say no, acknowledging their own needs and expectations, and their unique value systems. By collectively taking responsibility to inspire, teach and educate, we can provide young females with an opportunity to step into adulthood filled with hope and optimism.

In educational institutions, it's beneficial to introduce awareness, sexual-assault prevention and self-defence programmes. To find a suitable course provider, consider researching relevant programmes that are offered in your local area. When selecting an intervention programme for women, prioritize experienced instructors, and classes that address both the psychological and physical aspects of self-defence.

Ensure that the self-defence programme is not merely a by-product of a martial art discipline, as these programmes may introduce moves that appear impressive in videos but have little practical application in reality. Competent self-defence instructors understand this, and integrate various disciplines into their approach, combining techniques relevant to women in realistic self-defence scenarios. These techniques should include effective strikes, breakaway moves, and should address both standing and ground defence and offence. Verify the instructor's background and review their curriculum agenda before deciding to implement their programme in your institution.

If you're a female interested in joining a self-defence programme, search for educators with experience and approved credentials. Ideally, look for instructors with both practical knowledge in the field and a solid martial arts background, incorporating elements of striking and ground control. Apart from group classes, consider taking one-on-one sessions with a coach for a more personalized and focused approach.

When planning self-defence workshops for your company or institution, consider conducting a survey to identify the specific security concerns your staff may have. Share this information with the instructor who will be conducting the workshops so that they can tailor a bespoke course to meet the unique needs of your organization.

* * *

While physical training remains an important method in preparing for confrontation, I hope that this book has also expanded your understanding of self-defence more generally. When you become aware of all the psychological aspects which play a role in protecting your boundaries and safety, you can truly discover your strengths. You will understand the importance of building confidence and discovering ways in which to boost your self-esteem.

What's more, the words you say, the choices you make, and the energy you put out will have a ripple effect on others around you. Each time you assert yourself, you set an example of what it means to be a powerful woman. In doing so, you not only defend what is worth protecting, but also inspire other women to follow in your footsteps, forging a path toward strength, empowerment and positive change.

APPENDIX
SAFETY CHECKLIST

As we go about our daily lives, we should consider taking certain precautions. Below, you'll find a list of points to keep in mind, each accompanied by a checkbox.

- When heading out, I make sure to keep my phone fully charged, or carry a power bank with me. ☐

- I carry legal self-defence items with me, such as a defensive spray, or a personal safety alarm. ☐

- I don't accept drinks from strangers, unless they are served to me directly by the bartender. ☐

- I never leave my drink unattended in a bar, or at a social event. ☐

- When I'm by myself, I prioritize taking a taxi home after an evening out, especially when it's dark, or when I'm under the influence of substances. ☐

- I avoid wearing headphones when in an unsafe or unfamiliar environment, especially during dark hours or when I'm alone. ☐

- When walking alongside the road, I position my handbag on the side away from the road to deter potential snatch-and-grab incidents. ☐

- I always keep my bag closed in crowded spaces. ☐

- I usually carry a spare wallet with some petty cash to give out to potential muggers if approached or threatened. ☐

- I consistently research and respect local customs when travelling to unfamiliar destinations. ☐

- I am adept at dialling emergency services within seconds on my cell phone. ☐

- I have stored emergency contacts on my phone, and they are accessible to first responders. ☐

NOTES

NOTES

NOTES

NOTES